FREEDOM FROM
CANCER

FREEDOM FROM CANCER

THE AMAZING STORY OF VITAMIN B-17, OR LAETRILE

MICHAEL L. CULBERT

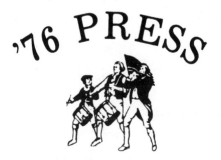

'76 PRESS

Seal Beach, California

Published by
'76 Press
P.O. Box 2686
Seal Beach, Calif. 90740

in cooperation with

**The Committee for Freedom of Choice
in Cancer Therapy, Inc.**
146 Main Street, Suite 408
Los Altos, Calif. 94022

Library of Congress Catalog Card Number 7643206
International Standard Book Number 0-89245007-X

MANUFACTURED IN THE UNITED STATES OF AMERICA

DEDICATION

To Bob and Bev,

Frank and Mo

because they are the

essence of liberty

And God said, Behold, I have given you every herb-bearing seed which is upon the face of all the earth, and every tree, in the which is the fruit of a tree yielding seed; to you it shall be for meat.

— GENESIS 1:29

In the history of science and medicine, there is no instance known of any chronic or metabolic disease that has ever been cured or prevented except by factors, water- or oil-soluble, normal to the diet and/or to the animal economy.

— DR. ERNST T. KREBS, JR.

ACKNOWLEDGMENTS

The author, who pleads guilty to being a journalist rather than a scientist, wishes to thank, effusively, all the principals in the story of vitamin B-17 (Laetrile) for their helpful guidance in developing this account — most particularly vitamin B-17's main pioneer, Dr. Ernst T. Krebs, Jr.; Bob Bradford, Beverly Newkirk, Frank and Maureen Salaman, and the staff of the Committee for Freedom of Choice in Cancer Therapy; Dean Burk, Ph.D., National Cancer Institute, cytochemistry division, who retired in 1974; my good friend Andrew R.L. McNaughton, founder and president of the McNaughton Foundation; Charles Gurchot, Dr. Krebs' mentor and an outstanding pharmacologist and Beardian; the courageous Doctors John A. Richardson, Stewart M. Jones and James Privitera, all of California; Ernesto Contreras, M.D., and Mario Soto de Leon, M.D., Tijuana, Mexico; and the pioneering Asian champion of vitamin B-17, Dr. Manuel Navarro.

The author also acknowledges that without the stimulus provided by California pharmacist Frank Cortese and the interest of William Loeb, New Hampshire newspaper publisher, this book would never have been written.

Nor would it have been written without the vital help of its major heroes and heroines — the men and women who spoke freely about their experiences with Laetrile as terminal cancer patients and who allowed me to come into their private lives so they could speak candidly and convincingly of their cases. To them, including the heroic battlers who later died, my eternal thanks.

Others played important roles by providing suggestions, clarifications, research, and related information. They include Wynn Westover, formerly with The McNaughton Foundation; Jean Blasdale, Berkeley, California; Malvina Cassese, San Francisco; Richard Ramella, a reporter for the *Independent-Gazette* of Richmond and Berkeley, California; my good friend Joaquin Relloma, San Jose, California, laboratory assistant and student of biology; David Rorvik of The Alicia Patterson Foundation; Mark McCarty, medical student at the University of California at San Diego; Charles Dahle, director of public information, American Cancer Society, California division; Robert M. Hadsell, Ph.D., Public Affairs Office, National Cancer Institute; John Steinbacher, International Association of Cancer Victims and Friends; and Betty Lee Morales and Lorraine Rosenthal, Cancer Contrrl Society; Jorge, Sergio, Gustavo, and Marco Del Rio and all the other Del Rio family members of Tijuana, Mexico, "los amigdaleros del norte;" and Donald Allison and matthew Jacobson, copyboys and ever-dependable and indispensable aids to a newspaper editor.

Any errors and omissions are entirely the fault of the author.

Contents

CHAPTER ONE

The Laetrile War

IN DECEMBER 1975, FEDERAL AGENTS, working with the smooth precision of a James Bond thriller, painstakingly traced a shipment of Mexican apricot kernel extract (brand name: Laetrile) in tablet and vial form to the homes of Donna Schuster and Donald Hanson, vitamin distributors in Rochester, Minnesota.

Once the merchandise had arrived, agents immediately seized the pair, confiscated records and materials, and said they were under arrest for conspiracy to smuggle "prohibited medicines."

ITEM: in this case the U.S. government — by admission in court affidavits — actually smuggled in its *own* Laetrile, had it first placed in and then seized it from the mails, specially packaged and specially shipped to the two Rochester, Minnesota homes.

Just three days earlier, twenty federal agents in thirteen undercover cars followed two Mexican citizens across half of California and waited while Robert W. Bradford, an electronics engineer on leave from Stanford University, met with a third Mexican and, according to the government's case, received a supply of the same material.

Bradford and two of the Mexicans were arrested and temporarily jailed on charges of conspiracy to smuggle.

Bradford's automobile was stolen by the government ("forfeited," in legal parlance), his bank account was frozen and personal papers were seized. Because the mild-mannered scientist also collects guns and had a Browning automatic in his possession, he was additionally charged with having a weapon while "in the commission of the offense."

ITEM: Bradford was the president of the then four-year-old Committee for Freedom of Choice in Cancer Therapy, Inc., a rapidly growing nationwide organization which originally had been established to help support a California physician and which had been saying for four years it would place American doctors in touch with apricot kernel extract, if the doctors so desired, and would place American cancer patients in touch with doctors who use the substance under its various names: vitamin B-17, Laetrile, amygdalin, nitriloside.

At about the same time, agents in New Jersey secured a court order to shut down — temporarily — a natural foods products distribution company in that state, alleging its distribution of "bitter food" tablets from West Germany (a kind of Laetrile also made from apricots) was tantamount to "endangering the health of the American public."

The following spring, federal agents, using approximately the same argument, raided a health food warehouse in Jacksonville, Florida and confiscated 470 pounds of apricot kernels. In both 1975 and 1976, federal and state agents visited a variety of health food stores in several states either issuing warnings about or actually confiscating supplies of apricot kernels the stores had on hand.

In May 1976, the original federal indictments against the Rochester pair and against Bradford were superseded by a "blanket indictment," one charging eight Americans, one Britisher, seven Mexicans and three Mexican business enterprises with participating in a vast apricot-kernel-extract distribution network. Federal agents worried out loud that the tentacles of the apparatus reached into every nook and cranny of a nation benevolently watched over by Big Brother.

There had, of course, been lesser skirmishes building up to the sweeping new indictments.

The Britisher (though brought up in Canada and the scion of a famed Canadian family), Andrew R. L. McNaughton, long the target of international wrath for promoting interest in and research concerning Laetrile, had been temporarily imprisoned in San Diego after crossing the Mexican-U.S. border with the ungodly amount of three-quarters of an ounce of apricot paste on his person.

Two years before, the government — using dubiously conducted tests in Arizona — had moved to ban from the shelves of health food stores and other outlets packages of Aprikern and Bee Seventeen, Laetrile-like products distributed as foods and, despite having been in circulation for many months and with millions of capsules sold, never having harmed a single person.

Along the U.S.-Mexican border at Tijuana-San Ysidro, a scenario was becoming more and more familiar as 1976 began:

American cancer patients, returning home with supplies of Laetrile from Mexico, where it is legal to use the stuff — as it is in two dozen other countries around the world[1] — were either forced to hide it, simply not to declare it, or to declare it and (depending on which U.S. Customs agent was doing the checking, and whether a supervisor happened to be looking) thus run the risk of having it confiscated.

One U.S. doctor crossing the border with a supply of the material was arrested. In California, the only state with specific anti-Laetrile statutes, Dr. John A. Richardson, a pioneering metabolic therapist who had boldly and openly used vitamin B-17 in his practice, and who had finally had charges of cancer quackery against him dismissed after being dragged through three trials, was re-arrested once again as part of the same "blanket indictment."

Federal, state and local police raided Dr. Richardson's Clinic in Albany, California, beat up a male medical aide, manhandled a nurse, and dragged Richardson's business manager off in handcuffs.

In 1975, state agents had twice arrested Dr. James Privitera of West Covina, California on a number of Laetrile connected charges; he had beaten most of them. California physician Stewart Jones, who had openly used Laetrile as vitamin B-17 in metabolic therapy, had been hauled before the State Board of Medical Examiners on a number of charges stemming from his daring use of an "unproven remedy" in treatment. He was acquitted on all but one allegation, but placed on probation. Later he was arrested on a Laetrile-connected charge after a state undercover agent, who swore under oath in a special hearing that she had been forced to sign her name to a false report in the matter, visited his office allegedly seeking help for cancer.

Were we seeing a James Bond thriller being enacted? Or was it something more Kafkaesque?

As the incredible pieces began falling together, the "Laetrile War" finally began catching the attention of the sluggish national media.

The entrapment of respected Minnesotans Donna Schuster and Don Hanson first received the spotlight of publicity, largely due to a battery of protest letters fired off by Bettie Gibson, editorial page editor of the Rochester *Post-Bulletin*. The *Post-Bulletin* was one of the few newspapers which, up to that time, had covered the Laetrile controversy with any objectivity. The journalist wrote everyone from President Ford to the Food and Drug Administration, and Senator Hubert Humphrey to local judges, demanding to know the hows and whys of the arrests of decent citizens for distributing vitamins.

Conservative columnist James Kilpatrick, aghast at the entrapments, turned out a series of piercing commentaries on what was clearly an outrage. Liberal Nicholas von Hoffman followed suit with radio commentary. The Hearst newspaper syndicate, and increasingly, large regional dailies, began giving relatively unbiased coverage to the matter.

What, they wanted to know, is going on?

What indeed?

That had been my question in 1970, when the Laetrile controversy was first made known to me, then the editor of the Berkeley, California, *Daily Gazette*, by a pharmacist, Frank Cortese, who insisted I interview cancer patients returning from Tijuana with credible accounts of incredible recoveries from their disease thanks to Laetrile.

The reader should know that I, as a journalist, was entirely skeptical of Laetrile when I first heard about it. But as I probed intermittently into a situation involving many Californians I was distressed to find that I could get no straight answer — and still can get no straight answer — to two overridingly important questions:

By what right does government interfere with the doctor-patient relationship and deny the doctor and the patient access to Laetrile (or anything else), particularly when that patient has been described as "terminal" and all "orthodox" remedies have failed? Indeed, why should honest Americans be treated as criminals and have to go underground or flee the country to secure a treatment which, at worst, is described as "worthless" and almost always admitted to be harmless?

The arrest in 1972 of Dr. John A. Richardson (see next chapter) turned out to be the decisive moment, both for the "Laetrile movement" and for me, personally, for since the "bust" occurred in the middle of the circulation area of the Brown newspapers (Berkeley and Richmond, California) and was instantly a major controversy, I could legitimately devote much professional time to the matter.

The net result of the arrest and the three trials which followed, where Dr. Richardson faced "cancer quackery" charges for open use of Vitamin B-17 (Laetrile) in the *metabolic treatment* of cancer, was the establishment of The Committee for Freedom of Choice in Cancer Therapy, Inc. At the time this was written, the Committee had grown to more than 400 chapters nationwide and involved 28,000 members, of whom 1100 were medical professionals (including about 800 medical doctors). At least fifty doctors were using Laetrile in their practice, whereas four years earlier perhaps five doctors in the country would admit to using the "unproven remedy."

In 1976, the Committee was leading the fight not only to vindicate and fully legalize Laetrile, but also the battle for freedom of choice in therapy across the board and to reduce government interference in medical practice. The Committee was holding seminars, symposias, showing Ed Griffin's combative filmstrip *World Without Cancer*, and also helping make available my first effort at investigative reporting on the Laetrile controversy, *Vitamin B-17: Forbidden Weapon Against Cancer* (New Rochelle: Arlington House, 1974). And it was holding doctors' workshops in which Laetrile therapy was the chief point of concern, but within the framework of a growing body of medical disciplines awkwardly and variously described as "metabolic therapy," "holistic medicine," "orthomolecular medicine," and "metabology."

The more vintage International Association of Cancer Victims and Friends (IACVF), originally established by a Laetrile-using cancer patient and which had manned the ramparts against bureaucratic harassment and medical blindness for more than a decade, remained very active in the fight for Laetrile, as did the Cancer Control Society and, more indirectly, the National Health Federation. All these advocacy and education groups, conducting campaigns on several fronts, were beginning to make their weight felt, individually and collectively, by 1976 — the same year in which the American Cancer Society, then riding high on an estimated $107 million budget, damned Laetrile as the "number-one problem in cancer quackery."

In 1976 — as in 1970, when I began my investigation — the "establishment" would not yield, not a millimeter, on the subject of Laetrile. Whether voiced by the American Medical Association, the American Cancer Society, the Food and Drug Administration, or state boards of public health, the argument against Laetrile was unequivocal: "not a shred of evidence" was the way FDA Commissioner Alexander McK. Schmidt put it at a science writers' seminar I attended in 1974. Laetrile was routinely denounced as "worthless," a "cruel hoax," a substance "consistently tested and retested in both man and animals with no effect." And yet:

— Thousands of Americans continued to flood the expanding Tijuana, Mexico, clinics, for legal treatment with the substance. Or, if they were more affluent, they went abroad, to West Germany or elsewhere, for Laetrile or equally "unorthodox" therapy. And, by 1976, several thousand more patients were being treated *within* the United States by hundreds of American physicians who were willing to risk peer review, or actual arrest (in California or along the border) in order to live up to their Hippocratic Oath. Of these thousands of American cancer patients, hundreds were rendering testimonials, many of them well supported with medical records, as to the efficacy of Laetrile and related treatment.

— Dean Burk, Ph.D., who retired in 1974 as head of the cytochemistry section, National Cancer Institute (which he had helped found), continued to claim that official statistics on the results of Laetrile animal tests, which were advanced by the "establishment" to "prove" the inefficiency of Laetrile, involved "misleading statements, red herrings, obfuscations and outright lies." He went so far as to attack officialdom's assessments of the NCI-Southern Research Institute statistics on Laetrile tests of Lewis lung cancer in mice by accusing "certain upper NCI administration spokesmen ... (of) scientific and immoral falsifications amounting to corruption in the sense of the Congressional Code of Ethics."

— A major controversy swirled at the prestigious Memorial Sloan-Kettering Cancer Center in New York, where, despite S-K directorate claims of "no efficacy" from Laetrile, *at least* seven sets of Laetrile tests in mice indicated the substance's capacity to block the metastasis (spread) of cancer in sick mice specially bred to develop mammary cancers. The S-K results fattened an admittedly lean but nonetheless significant list of tests at various places in the world where Laetrile *had* shown "a shred of evidence."

— More doctors than ever before were reporting *some* benefits from Laetrile (Vitamin B-17) therapy on patients. Clearly, a "shred of evidence" had occurred.

It seemed to me in 1976, as it had in 1970, that if there were just the *slightest* "shred of evidence" that Laetrile (amygdalin, vitamin B-17, nitriloside) had *any* effect in the treatment, let alone the prevention, of cancer, the substance should be as openly legal as aspirin is today — particularly if, as most of "orthodoxy" is quick to admit, the compound is harmless.

The law remained murky on the "legality" of Laetrile (see Chapter 2), but the substance has been treated *as if it were illegal,* which until recently was enough to keep cautious physicians away from it.

The reason Laetrile continues to be increasingly used, even on the black market, is quite simple:

It is the major "unorthodox" cancer therapy available at a time when, by every honest admission, the "orthodox" approach to cancer — indeed, the whole federally and privately funded "War on Cancer" — is failing.

The official statistics speak for themselves:

As of 1976, the projected death rate from cancer in the United States was more than 1,000 fatalities per day, or 370,000 per year — with the disease striking one out of every four Americans, killing one out of every six, affecting two of every three families, and constituting the number-one natural killer of children and the number-two natural killer of adults. More than 675,000 new cases of cancer were expected to be diagnosed in 1976, and at least 54 million Americans now living are expected to develop cancer in their lifetimes. These rates and figures were slightly higher in Great Britain, but the crude, awful fact is that in the "civilized" countries (for these facts and figures simply do not obtain in the "developing" or "uncivilized" countries) both the incidence of, and fatalities from, cancer have reached the highest levels in recorded history.

In 1976, the National Center for Health Statistics revealed the incredible fact that, with all of the 1975 health statistics compiled, cancer *alone* was showing a huge jump in the national death rate, while the nation's overall death rate was declining. In fact, while even the heart disease death rate was down in 1975 over 1973, and while the U.S. death rate had reached its lowest point in the nation's 200 years, cancer deaths had increased by a whopping 4.2 percent — or well over the most extreme cancer-death figures earlier estimated for 1975. The rate was far greater than at any time since World War II and represented an increase over another year (1974) in which the rate had, in turn, amazingly jumped by 1.9 percent over the previous year. Only suicide and murder joined cancer, the "natural" killer, as elements of the death rate which had increased in 1975 over 1973.

This is the backdrop against which the battle of statistics must be placed. First, because any rational view of this trend, which has been gaining every year since statistics have been kept, *must* indicate that what we're doing in an "orthodox" way to halt cancer simply isn't working.

"Establishment" medicine does its own juggling of statistics when it claims that, despite the truth of the above figures, cancer survival figures are better because the five-year survival rate for cancer has increased from one in five in the 1930s to one in three today. Such lobbying groups as the American Cancer Society point out that earlier diagnosis is a key to a better survival rate and argue that certain forms of cancer have shown marked increase in terms of survival rates. The above statements are true. But...

Daniel S. Greenberg, editor and publisher of *Science and Government Report*, stood the cancer establishment on its ear in 1975 when he reported that the actual survival rates have changed relatively little since 1955. The reason, he argued after an extensive investigation into cancer research and interviews with researchers themselves, may very well have been because the postwar introduction of antibiotics and blood transfusions helped reduce the toll from cancer surgery — that is, it was not that more patients were surviving *cancer* but that they were surviving the cancer *operations* which, in an earlier era, would have killed them.

While Greenberg's assessments came under instant fire from orthodoxy, it was quite another branch of the "establishment" that, perhaps unintentionally, backed him up. President Ford's Council on Environmental Quality reported in February 1976 that the incidence of cancer had more than doubled in the United States since 1900 and that there had been almost no improvement in survival rates since the 1950s. While noting that the greatest percentage of cancers seems somehow linked to the environment, the report added that the survival rate for stomach cancer remained at its 1950s level, for pancreatic cancer at its 1940s level, and the survival rate for lung cancer had risen only from 10 to 11 percent since the 1950s.

Greenberg's thorough analysis overturned a lot of misplaced optimism from the "establishment" — for example, its claimed giant strides in dealing with Hodgkin's disease, when this form of cancer accounts for only one percent of all cases.

Greenberg wanted to know where the research funds from the federally proclaimed "War on Cancer" were going, since press releases emanating from Washington (frequently paralleling the fund drive activity of the American Cancer Society), continued to speak almost exclusively of continuing research on methods which so far had not really dented the cancer incidence and mortality statistics: "heroic" surgery, radiation, and chemotherapy, the latter being the administration of poisons which have a radiation-mimmicking effect on the body and which led Laetrile and other non-toxic cancer therapy advocates to charge that as many *or more* cancer victims die from the *treatment* of cancer than from the disease itself.

Greenberg found many researchers who were willing to speak frankly — *if* guaranteed anonymity, a fact of life I myself encountered frequently during an on-again, off-again probe of the vitamin B-17 controversy.

An "internationally renowned expert on cancer statistics" at "one of the prime institutions of the cancer establishment" (wrote Greenberg) told him that: "There is very little in the way of new ideas, and when they do appear, the review committees that take a look at them are not receptive. They don't want to be contradicted. And the result is that people are reluctant to come forward with new ideas."

And what is the chief new idea?

"Prevention," said the anonymous expert. "Preventive medicine is always more effective than curative medicine, and now we have an immense number of clues about environmental origins of cancer . . . . But the establishment is made up of surgeons, radiologists, chemotherapists and virologists. Prevention has nothing to do with their training or outlook."

At the federally funded National Cancer Institute, a scientist told Greenberg: "Look, when you've got 10,000 radiologists and millions of dollars' worth of equipment, you give radiation treatments, even if study after study shows that a lot of it does more harm than good. What else are they going to do? They're doing what they've been trained to do. Like surgeons. They're trained to cut, so they cut."

A "physician who occupies a top administrative post" at another cancer research institution was equally blunt: "The problem is the closed mind of medicine," he said. "Orthodoxy prevails everywhere, and it's hard to get them to listen to a new idea. Remember that Papanicolaou (who devised the Pap test) published for 15 years before anyone would listen to him, but now you find the ACS extolling the virtue of the Pap test. I'm convinced that for some cancers the survival rates were better decades ago, but don't tell anyone I said that. The official line is that we're making a lot of progress."

By 1976, some $5 billion had gone into the "War on Cancer" — with no optimistic, tangible results. At the same time, the ACS had stepped up its diatribes against "cancer quackery" and the Laetrile War was in full swing.

"Orthodoxy" was still pursuing a 13th century approach to cancer — cutting it, burning it, or poisoning it. The results, extrapolated Dr. Dean Burk, with some liberalization, from National Cancer Institute statistics (see Chapter 11) are gruesome: a 7½ percent chance for a patient to survive for five years *if* he goes the cut-burn-or-poison route. While this was a somewhat misleading use of official statistics, it nonetheless underscored the reality that, with the exception of skin cancer, uterine cervical cancer in women, and a few rare cancer systems, the arrival in a clinic of a patient with clinical symptoms of cancer is virtually synonymous with a death sentence.

A University of California physiologist who studied cancer for 23 years released his own assessment of "orthodox" cancer treatment in 1975[3]:

Dr. Hardin B. Jones, of the UC Department of Medical Physics, said his studies "have proved conclusively that untreated cancer victims live up to four times longer than treated individuals." That is, *statistically*, one's probability of living longer and feeling better would be enhanced, following his discovery of a lump or bump, *if he opted to do nothing at all*! "Beyond a shadow of a doubt, radical surgery on cancer patients does more harm than good," Dr. Jones assessed. As for radiation treatments, "most of the time it makes not the slightest difference whether the machine is turned on or not."

The veteran physiologist argued that "orthodox" cancer therapy interferes with the body's natural defenses. "You see, it is not the cancer that kills the victim — it's the breakdown of the defense mechanism which eventually brings death."

One would imagine that with a public-private expenditure since 1971 of some $5 billion to track down the cause and cure of cancer, we would be geometrically closer to both. In fact, as I found time between running two newspaper staffs to learn all I could about cancer, and about Laetrile, I still imagined that was probably the case.

I was instructed on the "most modern thinking" about cancer while attending the sixteenth science writers' seminar of the American Cancer Society in 1974 in St. Augustine, Florida. Out of a sea of papers, presentations, and panel debates between the most qualified researchers, scientists, and investigators in the field this picture emerged:

• The specific cause or causes of the various human cancers are not known even though, runs majority opinion, the knowledge of cause or causes does not preclude the efficacy of certain treatments.

• There is no specific evidence that viruses actually cause cancer in humans, even though a number of viruses are associated with tumor systems and viruses seem to cause certain kinds of cancer in *in vitro* laboratory studies.

• It is not specifically known what causes a natural cell to become a malignant one.

• The vast incidence of cancer in this country is undoubtedly linked, at least in some way, to the "man-made" aspects of our "civilized" environment — with alleged carcinogenic factors abounding in the air we breathe and the food we eat. Yet the *modus operandi* of these carcinogens remains highly speculative.

• Chemotherapy, with or without selective surgery and radiation, remains the treatment of choice for the great majority of cancers — even though the survival levels for most metastasized cancer remain quite low. Some optimistic evidence was presented that combinations of chemo-therapy, rather than single agents, have far more effect on certain tumor systems. But even then prospects for cancer control are gloomy *unless* diagnosis and treatment are early.

• Emphasis still remains on treatment rather than on prevention, a reality pointed to by the most controversy-arousing researchers. It was pointedly remarked that an end to cigarette smoking would virtually eliminate lung cancer and upwards of 40 percent of cancer in American males.

For the writer, four items of major importance were forthcoming from the seminar of experts and the nation's top scientific writers:

• The viral theory of cancer, the presumption that most cancers are somehow caused by viruses, came under sharp attack by one researcher, whose contention — covered well by the rhetorical question: "Do viruses cause cancer or do cancers cause viruses?" — caused perhaps the sharpest single debate at the gathering.

• Increased interest in manipulating the body's immunity system as the first line of defense against cancer (or cancers — since conventional wisdom remains inflexible that cancer is a variety of at least 100 diseases without a probable single cause or probable single cure) was demon-strated and several researchers pointed to promising experiments in the field, their key premises being that disease is primarily a response by the host to disease-causing agents (pathogens) rather than the effect of the pathogens themselves, and that the breakdown and shoring up of the body's only partially understood immunity system and of its hormone system undoubtedly play dramatic roles in cancer.

• The key importance of nutrition in preventing and causing cancer was stressed by one researcher and provoked almost as great a controversy as did the attack on the viral theory of cancer. The same researcher decried the lack of nutritional training in the nation's medical schools and flatly stated: "Your doctor knows very little about nutrition."

• Newspaper writers from cities throughout the country reported pressure — amounting in some cases, they said, to "harassment" — from people demanding to know why vitamin B-17 (Laetrile) is not legal in this country, why human tests for Laetrile have not yet been authorized, why more people are not looking into the thousands of testimonials and claimed case histories of cancer control by Laetrile, and why desperate, terminal cancer patients may have no "legal" access to B-17 in this country. Why are such terminal patients forced to go sneaking off to Mexico or West Germany or some other country where they can procure the substance and be treated?

These four items are of more than passing importance to the vitamin B-17 story, for, as the reader will note, the essence of the vitamin B-17 approach to cancer rests on these assumptions: There is probably a single real *cause* of cancer, even though there are multiple "organizers" which can trigger off that single cause. Cancer is manifested, first, by a breakdown in the body's immunological system, and, second, by the absence of a vital food factor in the normal "civilized" diet. How diet impinges on the latter, and how it may affect the former, makes cancer, more than anything else, a specific vitamin-deficiency disease.

In the attack on the viral theory of cancer as an across-the-board explanation of the cause of the dread disease, Dr. Paul H. Black of the Harvard Medical School told the seventy science writers and editors that research is precise enough now so that "certainly caution must be voiced at the present time and theories that propose that all cancer inducing events operate via viral activation seem unwarranted and without substantial evidence."

The researcher on cancer viruses, a practicing physician, said that simply because viruses produced in the test tube may be inoculated in tissue and cause cancer tumors does *not* prove this is a natural chain of events in living organisms themselves. Indeed, he pointed out, viruses may result from tumors and certain viruses which may cause tumors outside the organism may not cause tumors in natural hosts. "Moreover, evidence is accumulating to indicate that the various inducing agents such as chemicals, radiation and hormones can cause a cancerous transformation in their own right," he added.

By *no* means was Dr. Black or any other researcher fronting for vitamin B-17 or were they in any way connected with the latter. But their points of view further opened the door to the possibility of the essential correctness of vitamin B-17 therapy.

Dr. Ernest L. Wynder, president of the American Health Foundation in New York, reported that there is "increasing evidence that nutrition plays an important role" among the environmental factors which are linked with cancer development. While drawing heavy fire from other scientists who have concentrated on the viral and/or other environmental but nondietary aspects of cancer induction, he did receive some support from Michigan State University physiologist and chemist Clifford W. Welsch, who, in discussing new research on hormone relationship to cancer, said: "There is no doubt that changes in one's eating habits could profoundly influence the endocrinological system" and thus affect the relationship of hormones to cancer. He added that "we really haven't tied in nutrition with carcinogens as we should."

Dr. Wynder, who challenged the American Cancer Society to focus far more attention on nutrition, said worldwide evidence of diet and cancer "relates largely to specific deficiencies or excesses in nutritional intake — an area which we may call 'malnutrition of the affluent,' already shown to be involved in cardiovascular diseases." In fact, he argued for use of the "prudent diet" already advanced for prevention of cardiovascular disease (reducing total fat calories from 43 to 35 percent, reducing cholesterol from 600 to 300 milligrams per day, eating no more than four eggs per week or red meat more than three or four times a week) for possible prevention of cancer. He noted that "as Japanese adjust to the American way of life they assume American dietary habits, develop American cholesterol levels and also acquire their rates of heart attacks." Specific studies have shown, too, that colon and breast cancer in Japan are more common among upper-income groups which have begun to "Westernize" their diets, he reported.

Dr. Wynder also pointed to the California study of Seventh-Day Adventists, whose collective lower meat consumption, nonsmoking and nondrinking he associated with lower rates of colon, pancreas, breast and prostate cancers than in the general population. He described as "aspects of nutrition and carcinogenesis that have been generally neglected in the past and deserve more attention" the apparent relationship between cancers of the colon and pancreas to cholesterol and bile acid metabolism, and the suspicion that hormone-related cancers may be linked to the effect nutrition appears to have on the constitution of cell membranes — and hence on the interrelation of hormones and hormone receptors. "I'm not saying nutrition is *the* cause of cancer, but *a* cause of major importance. It is not food additives I am talking about but excesses and deficiencies," he stressed.

At the seminar, the author asked Benno Schmidt, chairman of the President's Cancer Panel, why he had called on Sloan-Kettering to undertake preliminary tests on Laetrile, which received a rhetorical (but by no means substantive) shellacking at the gathering of experts and writers. The investment banker answered:

> *I have had more mail since I've been chairman on the subject of Laetrile than on any other single subject — virtually equal to all the mail on all subjects put together.*
>
> *There is a very considerable traffic in Laetrile. We know people are going to Mexico and other countries where Laetrile is legal. My only interest in Laetrile is that we find out for an absolute certainty what it does or does not do. A great many people think it doesn't do anything worthwhile and that it's something of a hoax to push this on the American people.*

At the conference, FDA Commissioner Alexander MacKay Schmidt (no relation to Benno Schmidt) was on hand to claim — in the face of reports that thousands of people report objective benefit from Vitamin B-17 — that "the fact that 10 to 15 thousand people believe that they've taken something that does them some good does not prove anything. We require some evidence, however slim, some rationale. We have traced down every lead we could find to try to determine some valid sign of efficacy (from Laetrile) and have not found any." And the ACS medical officer told the assemblage that recent National Cancer Institute studies on a specific kind of mouse tumor system treated with the substance had proved negative.

At the same time, in Washington, D.C., Dr. Dean Burk, still with the National Cancer Institute's cytochemistry division, released a lengthy, detailed rebuttal of the same study. Here are part of his conclusions, released on March 22, 1974:

> *I should make it clear that my analyses and conclusions differ diametrically from those of the SRI-NCI report where it is concluded that Amygdalin MF (NSC B900540, a form of Laetrile) "does not possess activity in the Lewis lung carcinoma system" ... or that "NSC B900540, either alone or in combination with NSC 128056 (beta-glucosidase), was inactive against established subcutaneous Lewis lung tumor when administered on the schedule of QD 7-15 days ..."*
>
> *In my opinion, the statistical analysis employed by the SRI was far from adequate, certain overriding biological considerations were neglected*

in the SRI-NCI report (though they should not have been), and, on top of this, certain upper NCI administrative spokesmen have been guilty of scientific and immoral falsifications amounting to corruption in the sense of the Congressional Code of Ethics.

In analyzing the experiments, the veteran biochemist said:

In Exp. 34, 54 and 63, any average grammar school student could, any SRI-NCI scientist should, and any sufficiently experienced statistician would, be able to see at a glance widespread evidence of Amygdalin MF efficacy, in terms of both absolute and percent positively increased median life span, most uniformly and notably so in the treatments with Amygdalin alone, but also in certain instances when beta-glucosidase was additionally given.

In the meantime, the continuing Sloan-Kettering tests on spontaneous mice tumors and the NCI-SRI ones on transplanted tumors cannot really be said to have addressed themselves to the primary, overriding concern: Is vitamin B-17 (Laetrile, amygdalin) effective or not in suppressing *human* cancer? Is it effective or not in preventing *human* cancer? No amount of animal tests can possibly answer either question. All of which makes the cover letter of the Test Laetrile Now Committee to President and Mrs. Nixon and the U.S. Congress, dated February 26, 1974, particularly poignant. Chairman Jay Hutchinson wrote:

Dear President and Mrs. Nixon and all Members of Congress:

The signatures of 8,000 Americans are enclosed. The total now stands at 43,000 who have signed the Test Laetrile Now Petition.

These 43,000 petitioners DEMAND that CLINICAL TESTING START NOW!

In only 43 days an equal number (43,000) Americans have died of cancer. Unquestionably, every one of these 43,000 cancer victims would have given their consent to clinical investigators and their own physicians to administer this non-toxic, pain-relieving *substance.*

Every day countless numbers of American cancer victims are forced by government edict to flee to foreign clinics to obtain Laetrile therapy.

How many cancerous mice must be saved by our scientists who are aware of Amygdalin's cancer-inhibiting power before one human life is saved, or significantly alleviated, within the borders of America?

What is your response, Mr. President, Mrs. Nixon, and Members of Congress, to the American cancer victim who has been told "there is nothing more we can do for you"?

We, the people, if not the physician, can do something — we are doing something to save our lives. We need your help. Now.

In 1974, Dr. Wynder and a few other duly credentialed scientists were virtually ignored when they pointed to the link between cancer and nutrition. But by 1976, oposition to this point of view was beginning to break down — thanks, in no small part, to *ad hoc* pro-natural foods groups, the "vitamin guerrillas" and the vitamin B-17 advocates, all of whom, in their own way, were making the case for *preventive* medicine and the paramount importance of diet to good health.

A mere $6 million of the $800 million National Cancer Institute budget for 1976 was earmarked for nutritional research and cancer, a move resisted by old-line researchers. And Robert A. Good, director of research at Memorial Sloan-Kettering Cancer Center, told Fairchild News Service[4] that he and his colleagues have "stumbled across one interesting idea — nutrition — as a means of manipulating the immune system," which, in turn, is the body's first line of defense against cancer.

"We found that we could increase or decrease immunity efficiency by varying the nutritional content of the diet," Good said. "In fact, we have doubled the life expectancy of a certain strain of mice through nutritional manipulation."

And such "establishment" organs as *Family Health/Today's Health* found much of interest and promise in the findings of a reduced cancer mortality and incidence among Seventh-Day Adventists, many of them in the Los Angeles area and thus exposed to the same pollutants and contaminants that many have suspected are involved with cancer induction. Though the Adventists' greatly reduced incidence of respiratory, mouth, pharynx, esophageal and bladder cancer have been linked primarily to their abstinence from cigarettes and alcohol, their lower rates in gastrointestinal and reproductive organ cancer appear to be linked to diet.[5]

Too, a report in January 1976[6] found "a much lower incidence of cancer among white residents of Utah" than among the American population as a whole. Again, religious proscription of alcohol and tobacco (72 percent of Utahans are Mormons) played an obvious role, but lower incidences of cancer not attributable to these factors remained "puzzling features" in the Utah cancer picture, the authors reported. Utahans developed even less colonic and rectal cancer than the Seventh-Day Adventists in California.

While the growing fields of orthomolecular medicine, preventive therapy, metabolic medicine (or "metabology") and "megavitamin therapy" were still being laughed at by the establishment, a few researchers were beginning to wonder — and were looking into the areas of vitamin therapy in cancer. In so doing, they were drifting closer and closer to the "quackery" world of Laetrile.

While "dramatic evidence" that Vitamin A helps reverse the effects of cancer was forthcoming from two American universities and a Swiss research center,[7] federal funds were refused for such investigations.

Dr. Linus Pauling, history's only two-time Nobel Prize winner, found it impossible to get federal funds for his research in treating cancer with Vitamin C, despite growing evidence of Vitamin C efficacy in cancer.

But the tide was turning, slowly but perceptibly. A medical revolution stressing prevention over treatment, and focusing more attention on diet, was dimly visible over a horizon littered with the human carnage representing the wholesale failure of Western medicine to apply its allopathic nostrums to degenerative disease.

As we shall see, vitamin B-17's threat to cancer, and the threat of holistic medicine itself to the overlap of vested interest in allopathic medicine, expensive and toxic drugs, radiation, surgery, the "health-care delivery" industry, the international drug cartel and the food processing industry, may explain much of the opposition to the extract of apricot kernels.

In learning to separate the wheat from the chaff in the Laetrile controversy, which began assuming the proportions of World War III by 1976, I learned what the proponents of Laetrile actually were saying and claiming, in distinction to what the "establishment" opposition *said* they were claiming and saying.

First off, Dr. Krebs himself and the inner core of what may be called the "Laetrile movement" were *not* peddling the need for everyone to go out and buy the product Laetrile, in either tablets or vials. What they were saying — what *we* are saying, since I moved from skeptic to objective observer to advocate — is that proper diet is very likely *the* way to prevent cancer from occurring in the first place. And that the primary operative factor is that massively abundant substance variously referred to as cyanophoric glycosides, beta-cyanogenetic glucosides, nitriloside, or vitamin B-17. This food factor has been removed from the basic Western diet both by habit (switching from millet to wheat as a basic cereal, for example; spitting out fruit seeds instead of chewing them, for another) and by the methodology of food processing. We have been left, in the West, with a diet of processed, tampered-with foods almost totally devoid of vitamin B-17 — and yet, as you will read in the recipes in the appendices of this book, there are many ways, with very little trouble, to restore vitamin B-17 to your diet.

Secondly, the Laetrile advocates are saying that once there *is* clinical cancer, and while many forms of therapy may be used to "reduce a tumor," tumor reduction itself is no more a valid criterion for actually "treating" cancer than is the treatment of the *symptoms* of syphilis a genuine attack on the disease itself. The Laetrilist position is that, by and large, vitamin B-17 (in the form of injectable and tablet Laetrile) *and in conjunction with other vitamins, enzymes, dietary change and detoxification,* is *the* most biologically rational and reasonable approach to a cancer crisis. The underlying theory is that it is *not* cancer, but basic metabolism, which is being treated, and that it is the body — not the doctor — which ultimately corrects the disease condition.

Wild claims have *not* been made for Laetrile, as a careful perusal of the following pages will demonstrate. Laetrile is *not* a "mysterious cancer cure-all," as the opposition says Laetrilists are claiming. The most extreme claim made for Laetrile therapy is that it will "control" (but not cure) cancer just as insulin controls (but does not cure) diabetes. The growing evidence of Laetrile therapy around the world supports the following claims, despite the enormous propaganda campaign raised in the United States against it:

Laetrile therapy will *at least* provide palliation (or total elimination) of cancer-connected pain in *most* cases; *most* Laetrile patients report a general improvement in the sense of well-being, improvement in appetite, and gain in weight — all of these things being abundant blessings, particularly for the dying and desperate who represent the 85 to 90 percent of patients in North America who turn to Laetrile as a last-ditch therapy. Also widely reported are reductions or elimination of the offensive odor connected with many cases of cancer, and prolongation of life even when the patient ultimately expires.

In pursuing Laetrile testimonials across the country, I learned of case after case in which cancer, while by no means "cured," was indeed stabilized for long periods of time apparently due to Laetrile and its ancillary therapy. I know of other cases in which the palpable symptoms of cancer continued under B-17 therapy but the patients felt better while even certain of ultimate death — and they blessed Laetrile for feeling better. There was of course that exciting small percentage — about 5 percent — in which all palpable symptoms of cancer vanished entirely under Laetrile therapy. (Orthodoxy consistently appends the tag "spontaneous remission" to this cluster of testimonials.)

Most important of all, Laetrile can be taken in large doses with no apparent toxic side-effects, so totally in contrast with the chemotherapeutic poisons of "approved" therapy, with their sequelae of falling hair, horrible nausea and continual malaise. And the injections and tablets of Laetrile are not, apparently, contraindicated in "orthodox" therapy, although the hard Laetrilist position is that "orthodox" therapy should be avoided as much as possible.

But above and beyond the scientific skirmishes over Laetrile are the much graver questions:

Since it is admittedly harmless, *why* is Laetrile being suppressed? How dare politics enter the field and disrupt the doctor-patient relationship?

You will read here of the earlier battles of "unorthodoxy" versus the "establishment." Luckily, for the first time in medical history in the United States, "unorthodoxy" is on the march to victory — and this because the Laetrile issue became wedded to the political and moral issue of "freedom of choice."

By 1976 — symbolically enough, America's Bicentennial Year — important breakthroughs had occurred:

• In California, where Laetrile was most vigorously and viciously suppressed, "freedom of choice" advocates, usually skippered by "Laetrile lawyer" George Kell, had won a dozen cases for physicians and other citizens ensnared by California's anti-Laetrile statutes, even though the Laetrile "crimes" were advanced from misdemeanor to felony status. The cases represented courtroom victories for the concept of metabolic therapy and the freedom to choose alternative therapies.

• The State of Alaska, spurred by vigorous efforts of Committee for Freedom of Choice in Cancer Therapy, Inc. chapters, became the first State in the Union to pass a "freedom of choice" law allowing the use of vitamin B-17 in therapy there. The law was passed on June 21, 1976, despite last-minute pressure from the Food and Drug Administration and misleading propaganda by the Alaska Medical Board.

• Minnesota Senator Hubert Humphrey, responding to the national furor raised over the entrapment arrests of two of his constituents, Rochester vitamin distributors Donna Schuster and Don Hanson, called for an FDA hearing on Laetrile "in light of continued favorable comment on its effectiveness by users."

• Western Oklahoma U.S. District Court Judge Luther Bohanon had issued 18 court orders allowing "terminal" cancer patients in the United States to receive their supplies of Laetrile without interference from the FDA, which, he ruled, had long since abrogated its right to rule in the Laetrile matter. The federal government appealed the judge's rulings.

• Congressman Steve Symms of Idaho had introduced a bill to overturn the "efficacy" clause of the Food, Drug and Cosmetic Act Amendment of 1962, which has been a key factor in the blocking of the access of the public to needed substances.

How had it happened? What lay behind the Laetrile War?

It is, indeed, an incredible story — a newsman's delight, so to speak, which explains how I got into it in the first place. What follows is the full story of Laetrile (vitamin B-17), one of the most multi-faceted controversies of this century.

CHAPTER TWO

Of Mice and Men and Cancer

IN JUNE 1972, NEWS MEDIA in the San Francisco Bay Area were alerted through friendly sources in the Alameda County district attorney's office that a newsworthy "bust" was in the works. Sure enough, state and local officers, armed with warrants charging Dr. John A. Richardson of Albany, California, and two of his nurses with multiple violations of the state's "cancer quackery" statutes, burst into the doctor's clinic.

Using what the respected physician described as "Gestapo tactics," officials confiscated his records and arrested him and two nurses, because, said the state, they had dispensed an illegal substance called Laetrile to cancer patients. One of the "patients" turned out to be an undercover agent. And Laetrile for use in cancer therapy is expressly forbidden by sections of the California health and safety codes.

As it turned out, Dr. Richardson proved to be the wrong man arrested in the wrong place at the wrong time on the wrong charge. Dr. Richardson was an outspoken member of the John Birch Society. And neither he nor any of his friends intended to back away from a good fight. The Richardson arrest marked the explosive entrance into the vitamin B-17 controversy of numerous Birchers, many of them grouped in a complex of ad hoc committees collectively known as the Committee for Freedom of Choice in Cancer Therapy, Inc.

Between the time they were originally set up as support groups for the Richardson trials and June 1976, the ad hoc committees or "chapters" had proliferated to more than 400 across the country. They represented almost every state in the Union, and had enlisted more than 28,000 members (including 800 medical doctors and 300 other medical professionals).

The organization, led by electronics engineer Robert W. Bradford, previously employed at the Stanford Linear Accelerator and later indicted on smuggling charges, swiftly became a major force in the advocacy of vitamin B-17 (Laetrile) therapy, metabolic medicine, and the need to remove governmental interference from the practice of medicine. The four-year growth of about 100 chapters per year paralleled the rising tide of the Laetrile controversy. The movement received added impetus from the International Association of Cancer Victims and Friends (IACVF), led by writer John Steinbacher, which also organized units in Canada and fought for recognition of a wide range of "non-toxic" cancer therapies.

A split-off group, the Cancer Control Society, under the tutelage of nutritionist Betty Lee Morales, also joined the battle. Independent pro-Laetrile, pro-"unorthodoxy" groups sprouted across the country with, if you'll pardon the expression, cancerous velocity. All of them were springing to the defense, in one way or another, of the badly buffeted Laetrile — the brand name for the purified, crystallized, freeze-dried form of the compound amygdalin.

The arrest of Dr. Richardson thus began a decisive turnabout in Laetrile's tangled history — indeed, it set the stage for an historic first in American medical history, when "unorthodoxy" seized the offensive.

Laetrile, which had *de facto* legal acceptance in two dozen other countries, had been proscribed from interstate shipment and sale in the United States for a decade. Since 1963 it had been specifically prohibited from use in cancer therapy, on humans, in California — where it had been pioneered.[1]

The legal situation surrounding Laetrile became a snare-laden semantical and jurisdictional headache. To begin with, the FDA proscription against Laetrile was not a written ban *per se* and the substance did *not* appear on any list of officially banned items. As of 1976, the only federal "law" against Laetrile was not a law at all, but a regulatory guideline from the FDA, an "import alert" dated October 7, 1974, whereby federal officials (usually Customs agents) were told that both Laetrile *or any Laetrile-like product* was either an "unlicensed new drug" or "adulterated in that it is a food additive that is unsafe within the meaning of" federal codes. If Laetrile could be construed as unsafe, then it *could* be brought within the purview of the FDA's somewhat murky jurisdiction.

But what if Laetrile, the extracted form of amygdalin from apricot kernels (or similar sources), were neither a new drug, an old drug, nor an unsafe or adulterated food additive? What then?

This is precisely the case advanced by Laetrile adherents, particularly since the vitamin nature of amygdalin and the range of compounds variously called cyanophoric glycosides, beta-cyanogenetic glucosides, or nitrilosides, was not elaborated until the 1960s nor popularly published until 1970.[2] It remained for Dean Burk, Ph.D., the salty biochemist with the National Cancer Institute who rose to do battle for Laetrile *within* the "establishment," to further expand on the vitamin nature of the nitrilosides. The point became one of enormous legal significance, quite aside from its scientific controversy: If Laetrile was, in effect, simply a vitamin (or even construed as a "food additive" — rendering it a food, since any part of a food *is* a food), then its use was outside the jurisdiction of the FDA. This is particularly true if no precise therapeutic claims were made for it. The vitamin-versus-drug battle became doubly important after the passage, in 1976, of the Proxmire Law which effectively got the FDA out of the business of regulating vitamins.

Even if Laetrile were construable as a drug (which it might be under the most generous application of semantics), then the fact it had been known in its natural form (amygdalin) for well over a century, and even therapeutically used a century before (see Chapter 5), hardly made it a "new drug." If it were not a drug, new or old, then it did not need a license and could not be under the jurisdiction of the FDA.

To repeat, as of 1976 there was *no* federal "law" against Laetrile, only the attempt to keep it out of interstate shipment and sale by FDA when presented as a *product*. California had passed vigorous anti-Laetrile statutes, but these bore solely on the use of the substance to treat cancer in human beings. A string of court cases in 1974 and 1975, beginning with the Richardson trials, questioned both the State's official definition of cancer and whether a vitamin somehow used in its management could be regarded as a "drug" used to "treat" the disease. *If* amygdalin, as vitamin B-17, were being given in metabolic treatment along with other vitamins, minerals and enzymes, and if the metabolism itself were doing the "treating," then the use of Laetrile could not be defined as a "treatment for cancer." While the "establishment" contended this argument was a convenient way to get around state law, the argument did correctly express the viewpoint of the rapidly growing field of metabolic medicine — namely, that cancer is a local manifestation of a systemic or metabolic disease, and that it is the body itself which does the "treating." The Laetrile physicians of the 1970s almost entirely make that distinction: Laetrile, as vitamin B-17, is part of a nutritional or metabolic treatment of the whole person, not an attack on tumors.

But in 1972, when there was but a handful of physicians who dared to use Laetrile, the arrest of Richardson was based on the contention the doctor was using an "unproven" or "quack" cancer "cure" in his practice. A few doctors had run afoul of such anti-quackery regulations in earlier years. But unlike some other physicians leaned on by Big Brother, the independent-minded Richardson fought back. The immediate reaction to his arrest was the rapid spread of the Committees for Freedom of Choice in Cancer Therapy.

The existence of the ad hoc committees brought forth hundreds of new testimonials to add to the thousands that had been accumulating since the early 1950s. All attested to Laetrile's dramatic effects, which ranged from relief of pain (the single most overwhelming symptom reported) to spectacular regressions of tumors and even complete recoveries. What had been a simmering hostility between proponents of Laetrile and entrenched medical orthodoxy and governmental bureaucracy erupted into open war.

Supplies of Laetrile manufactured in Tijuana, Mexico — where thousands of American patients had gone seeking treatment since 1963 — were somewhat curtailed in 1973 by a crackdown on alleged smugglers of the substance. Letter-writing campaigns had brought the matter to the attention of the Nixon administration. Newspaper articles and television reports turned the Laetrile controversy into a national news story. While officialdom continued claiming there were absolutely *no* beneficial effects from Laetrile treatment and insisted that Laetrile was a "worthless" extract of the apricot kernel, more and more persons stepped forward with credible case histories of Laetrile's efficacy. Mixed results from tests at the prestigious Memorial Sloan-Kettering Cancer Center served as a stimulus for more demands to "Test Laetrile Now!" and to prove that "Laetrile Works — You Bet Your Life!" — the slogans adopted by pro-Laetrile organizations in 1972.

Dr. Richardson readily admitted he had dispensed Laetrile to his patients — but only, he argued, as vitamin B-17 and as part of a general megavitamin therapy. He insisted that such usage was legal under California law, since amygdalin is recognized as useful in metabolic deficiency.

A tantalizing legal question thus arose: if it were legitimate to use amygdalin (the chemical, generic term for Laetrile or vitamin B-17) in megavitamin therapy, then a hole had been poked in the patchwork of laws making the substance illegal in the treatment of cancer. The case became a landmark one and interest in it grew with the velocity of a fulminating neoplasm.

The long, involved court process got under way in the municipal jurisdiction of Berkeley, California — perhaps the most innovative, unorthodox and "anti-establishmentarian" city in the United States. Its very name conjures up cliches ranging from "Athens of the West" (with love) to "Peking East" (with hatred) and its institutions had been sorely tested by activism and revolt since the onset of the Free Speech Movement in 1964 at the University of California.

Having covered explosive, radical Berkeley since 1964, as a newsman I was particularly interested in the theatrics that might accompany the court appearances of a conservative Bircher like Dr. Richardson. The courthouse in downtown Berkeley had been for years the scene of many demonstrations and near riots, ranging back to the FSM and Vietnam Day Committee periods. Its chambers had teemed with hundreds of the mostly young, mostly hip, mostly radical communards in Berkeley sometimes called "the counter-culture" or, by the *Berkeley Daily Gazette*, the "anarchoradiboppers."

When Dr. Richardson appeared for arraignment and for his first trial, hundreds of individuals showed up to view the proceedings. They included not only "streets" but, in the Berkeley parlance, "straights" — clean-cut men and traditionally dressed women. No placards, no chanting, no revolutionary slogans, no disruptions from this assembly.

For months the Richardson case moved in and out of court, ultimately landing in Alameda County Superior Court, where the doctor, convicted on five counts of violating health and safety codes, switched his attorneys and his attack. A legal snarl ensued as the case became a pitched courtroom confrontation between the ever-growing legion of Laetrile supporters and defenders of the State's rigid legislation against its use. This was a bellwether case that could break nationally the federally imposed ban on the use of the substance in cancer therapy.

In 1973, the appellate division of the Alameda County Superior Court reversed the convictions of Dr. Richardson and nurses Margaret Grosch and Charlotte Anderson on a series of technicalities. A new trial was ordered. The second trial began in Berkeley-Albany Municipal Court; in the interim various counts had been dropped and others were added. The Albany physician continued, during the whole period, to use Laetrile in his general megavitamin therapy.

After three weeks, the second trial ended in a hung jury; the jurors noted that a majority of them favored outright acquittal. A United States federal judge refused to hear the case until Richardson and his attorneys had exhausted all state-level legal alternatives, and a third trial was ordered for 1974.

It, too, resulted in a hung jury — but this time the charges were dismissed. What had happened was that Dr. Richardson had been dragged through *three* misdemeanor trials, with all of the powers of the State against him, without a single conviction.

But the case didn't stop there, of course. Since Richardson had become the first California physician to beat the California Laetrile Laws, powerful forces went into gear to increase the anti-Laetrile statutes to felony status, and to find some way — any way — to "get" Richardson.

How else explain the long and seemingly systematic pattern of harassment that then ensued? The California doctor, who continued, boldly and openly, to use vitamin B-17 in his practice, became a target for wrath of all kinds: the Internal Revenue Service was salivating to get the Albany physician and came within a whisker of attaching his home in nearby Orinda. Other federal agencies moved against Richardson for one thing or another; and state officers fanned out across California attempting to find former patients and relatives of former patients who would file suits against him.

Not until the group indictments on "conspiracy to smuggle" in 1976 was Richardson again arrested — and this occurred when he appeared in Sacramento to testify in favor of "freedom of choice" bills then being heard by the Assembly. While he was arrested in Sacramento, his clinic was raided in Albany, a nurse there pummeled and an aide beaten up.

The Richardson trials in 1972-1974 were the center of attention as a Laetrile propaganda war raged on both sides. During this time the California physician continued to stump the state and the nation lecturing not only on metabolic therapy and B-17 but also on the fantastic encroachments by government into the medical profession.

The Food and Drug Administration, the National Cancer Institute, and the American Cancer Society were repeatedly asked why Laetrile was not legal. They issued their customary denunciations, most of them based on an early series of tests done in California in 1953. The line was united and recurring: there is no substantive evidence that Laetrile has anti-tumor effects; testimonials don't mean very much; what's more, Laetrile might be dangerous.

The pro-Laetrile groups and those interested in natural foods and nutrition denounced the FDA, the American Medical Association, and the American Cancer Society as either blind or malicious or both.

The situation was tailor-made for hard-nosed conservatives: the crackdown on Laetrile, Birchers and non-Birchers claimed, was fresh evidence of a conspiratorial government involved with pharmaceutical monopolies or engaged in an insidious scheme to allow government to "discover" Laetrile as a cancer cure and use it as a pretext for socializing medicine.

The extremist positions at both ends — one, that Laetrile is utterly worthless and merits no further time and effort; the other, that Laetrile and the theory behind it constitute the final, definitive answer to cancer — obscured, as usual, the more centrist reality. Obviously, there is something to Laetrile, and the growing wave of evidence makes a compelling case for facing this fact without assuming Laetrile is the total answer or that all opposition to Laetrile has an identical interest in its suppression.

About the same time the ad hoc Committees for Freedom of Choice began operating, the California-based Test Laetrile Now Committee was busily circulating petitions to then-President and Mrs. Richard Nixon, urging them to intervene with the FDA to "clear" Laetrile, a substance pioneered almost a quarter-century before, for tests on humans. This was in alignment with the view that somehow Laetrile *could* go through normal FDA channels and eventually come up with a testing license. Hard-core Laetrilists questioned whether that move was really necessary, since Laetrile's use in two dozen other countries, they thought, constituted "human tests" galore. By the time the petition campaign — headed by San Francisco insurance salesman Jay Hutchinson, who had been controlling his lymphosarcoma with Laetrile for two years — had ended, 43,000 signatures had been gathered. The signatures came primarily from persons who were using or had used the substance, and from their families and friends.

In December 1973 Hutchinson and Cancer Victims United wrote the Nixons to complain that the United States Customs Department "is preventing life-maintaining supplies of Laetrile from reaching us here in the United States. Please issue a Presidential Decree of Mercy . . . so that those of us patients already taking Laetrile may continue the effective control of cancer we have established within ourselves using this substance." It went on to state that "the FDA and the Customs Department people have apparently agreed that the best way to eliminate the favorable case histories of the control of our cancers by Laetrile is to stop all supplies, thus depriving us of this life-sustaining substance."[3]

Indeed, as Customs officials told Frank Winston, who was at the time West Coast editor of the *National Tattler*, eleven people had been arrested on the California-Mexican border between August and the end of 197, as smugglers of Laetrile. Most were Mexican nationals, and the arrests were carried out because the size of the supplies seized indicated a "commercial" intent. Usually, however, customs officials looked the other way when American cancer patients recrossed the border from Tijuana with their own personal supplies of the substance. The standard practice was to allow them to cross without difficulty if they could produce a prescription for the medicine, which achieved full legal status in Mexico in 1973.

Some spectacular cases of Laetrile efficacy came to light in 1974, indicating early and effective response to the treatment.

An eighteen-year-old Plainview, Minnesota youth who had been diagnosed with what had begun as testicular cancer, stunned Minnesota television audiences with his case history, which had involved the prestigious Mayo Clinic. He was diagnosed first at a Minnesota hospital, then underwent exploratory surgery at Mayo. He was told, according to his parents, that he would need cobalt treatment. His mother recalled that the physician told him of a host of bad side effects from cobalt and indicated he might have only a year to live even with the treatments. That was in early 1972. His parents had already heard of the Laetrile treatment and knew that the only relatively close place to procure it was Tijuana.

The young man went to Tijuana for treatment in January 1972 and was there until May 1972. He underwent the standard Laetrile injections at the Contreras clinic and was also given enzymes and a strict diet. He returned home and continued taking the Laetrile tablets until September 1972. All cancer systems vanished. Subsequent checkups by United States doctors, his parents insisted, showed him to be cancer-free. One of his original physicians was quoted as saying: "We are at a loss to explain what happened." Under the usual Laetrile treatment, a cancer victim is assumed cancer-prone for the rest of his life and the usual procedure is to keep him on a Laetrile maintenance intake for his lifetime, much as a diabetic must stay on insulin. The young man "felt fine" when I talked to him in January 1974.

Such results came as no surprise to several solidly credentialed clinicians around the world where Laetrile therapy is legal (if not necessarily preferred). Cancer and other therapy with amygdalin was reported in the Soviet Union in the 1970s, and Yugoslavia was known to have its own amygdalin-processing laboratory.

The scientific controversy around Laetrile, fought in medical journals and occasionally in the press, sputtered on intermittently for years. It was the raid on Dr. Richardson's office that made Laetrile hot news once again — and also convinced me to get cracking on untangling the full, incredible story of a banned substance that reliable doctors and scientists contended was a cancer palliative at worst, and perhaps at best an outright control (not a cure) for the dread Big C.

Instantly, the Richardson case not only triggered off the swift development of ad hoc committees; it also wrought a strange coalition between the hard-right traditionals and the hard-left counter-culture, a phenomenon most noticeable in ever-against-the-grain Berkeley. It was not uncommon in 1972 to see many psychedelically painted campers and panel trucks plying the streets of Berkeley, San Francisco, and other Bay Area cities bearing such seemingly disparate bumper stickers as "Vote McGovern" and "Test Laetrile Now!" The marching slogan "Laetrile Works — You Bet Your LIfe!" could be seen on a hippie van and a Cadillac.

Indeed, the natural-health-nutritional-therapy wing of the back-to-nature counter-culture found in the plight of Laetrile and of the good Birch doctor a sympathetic overlap with the straight world. Both sides could cheer as the Albany physician went before 1,100 people in San Francisco's Fairmont Hotel in early 1973 to rip the "tinseled tones and lilting lies" of "medical bureaucrats" and to scorn the "tinhorn megalomaniacs safely ensconced in the federal bureaucracy who harass men and women who are continuing to do their duty to God, family, and country."

Dr. Richardson, a handsome and articulate new hero of the Laetrile cause, stumped the state and the nation proclaiming the vitamin B-17 gospel to an ever-increasing audience. Cancer, he told anyone who would listen, is primarily a specific vitamin-deficiency disease. A substance called vitamin B-17, occurring naturally in more than 1,200 plants, vegetables, and grasses (and not recognized as a vitamin by the FDA, the American Medical Association, and the American Cancer Society), is the specific vitamin that provides the body's essential backup defense against cancer. The incidence of cancer is epidemic in many civilized countries because some natural vitamins have been removed from processed foods.

The corollary, so heartening to anti-establishmentarians of all stripes and which helped to weld the strange coalition of Laetrile advocates, is essentially this: The medical elite and the corresponding government bureaucracy are somewhere between pervasively naive and criminally irresponsible in disallowing the "unofficial" clinical evidence for the efficacy of vitamin B-17. Meanwhile, a mammoth "cancer industry" — expressed in hospitals, surgery, radiation, treatment, and highly toxic chemotherapy — has become a multi-billion-dollar annual operation. And all this while up to 370,000 Americans per year are dying of cancer — a thousand a day — and cancer fatality levels have reached the highest point in history.

The Richardson arrest and subsequent litigation were by no means isolated incidents in the lengthy, disjointed, on-again, off-again story of Laetrile — a word coined by San Francisco biochemist Ernst T. Krebs, Jr. to define both the processed form of amygdalin and a whole class of natural substances, of which amygdalin is the most medically prominent representative. Krebs and his father, the late Ernst T. Krebs, Sr., M.D. (who died cancer-free at age ninety-three), had run afoul of the FDA and state laws on several occasions because of their work in developing and manufacturing Laetrile.

In February 1971 state agents arrested Krebs, Jr. and four others, including a woman who ran a rooming house catering to Mexico-bound cancer patients, on a variety of state health-law violations. The biochemist, about whom much more later, told me the quintuple arrests preceded the airing of an NBC television program on Laetrile. "We know the orders come down from on high," the thick-jowled scientist who devoted most of his college life and his entire professional life to the conquest of cancer said. "As long as what we're doing doesn't receive public attention, they let us alone. But within twenty-four to forty-eight hours of major publicity, the FDA moves vigorously and viciously."

In May 1971 the California Department of Public Health actually tried to secure a court order that would have prohibited the publication of articles suggesting the efficacy of Laetrile. Happily, a superior court judge bounced the case out of court as a violation of the First Amendment. This decision set the stage for champions of vitamin B-17 to hold major conventions throughout 1973 — attended by up to 1,500 people each — during which the alleged benefits and controlling properties of the substance were discussed.

Earlier, on March 12, 1970, the Pennsylvania Health Department swooped down on a meeting of the Harrisburg Natural Food and Health Association after the movie *Laetrile, Nature's Answer to Cancer* was shown. The film was confiscated and the association president, Bruce Butt, arrested. Urged by officialdom to plead guilty, Butt refused. The National Health Federation stepped in to give him a legal hand and two years later he was exonerated of the "cancer quackery" charges leveled against him. Arrests of several members of the International Association of Cancer Victims and Friends followed the same year.

Inasmuch as the FDA had refused in 1963 to allow interstate shipment of Laetrile, and inasmuch as the official line, developed ten years before, was that the substance was worthless, and inasmuch as many state health codes contain provisions against the use or advocacy of unofficial cancer treatments, doctors who dared use or advocate Laetrile were quite literally risking their careers. Since terminal cancer patients in the United States were denied access to this alternative treatment, and since American doctors risked heavy penalties if they were in any way involved with the Krebs discovery, it was no mystery that many patients began seeking the nearest source of open, legal Laetrile treatment — Tijuana, Mexico. More affluent terminal cancer patients headed for Dr. Hans Nieper's facilities in Hannover, West Germany, where general therapy in which amygdalin played a central role was available.

Not until Dr. Richardson became involved in Laetrile therapy, and was arrested for his efforts, did the public learn that a handful of American physicians were prepared to risk their professional lives by making the illegal compound available in this country. At the beginning of 1974, Dr. Richardson told me he had treated more than 750 patients with his megavitamin therapy that included vitamin B-17; his actions were an open challenge to the California Health and Safety Code statutes banning the use of "laetriles" (specifically, amygdalin and prunasin) in cancer treatment. Also by 1974, Atlanta urologist Larry McDonald, who became a believer in Laetrile after attending a San Francisco seminar on the subject a year before, said he had treated 80 patients with the substance. Dr. McDonald went on to become a United States Congressman, an outspoken champion of both vitamin B-17 and "freedom of choice" — and the target of as much harassment as could be thrown at a congressman.

But a key legal question remained, for the time, unanswered: Does a terminal, dying cancer patient *not* have the right to access to a substance, however opposed it may be by the American medical establishment? Some states seemed to say he does have that right. But in California, birthplace of the development of Laetrile and discovery of vitamin B-17, the "drug" remained vigorously opposed. And, as far as federal law was concerned, Laetrile remained illegal for interstate sale and shipment.

As to the matter of the rights of a dying cancer patient, one of Dr. Richardson's first attorneys, the colorful General Clyde Watts of Oklahoma, came up with a fresh idea. He entered a suit against federal authorities on behalf of an Oklahoma terminal cancer patient denied access to Laetrile, a constitutional class action suit "on behalf of all people dying of cancer." Though Watts' first client died before the suit was filed, the combative barrister filed the suit on behalf of several other patients, including Kansan Glen Rutherford, whose full recovery on the Laetrile program became a *cause celebre*. A United States District Court Judge in Oklahoma agreed with his attorneys that the FDA had no right to interfere with his access to vitamin B-17. Clyde Watts died in a plane crash while his series of terminal patient-clients were securing court orders allowing them access to Laetrile. But as of 1976 more patients were opting for the court-order approach even while the United States government, stung by the United States District Court ruling, appealed the decision.

A second Richardson attorney, George Kell of Modesto, California, decided to argue the Richardson case in part on the basis of the Supreme Court decision in *Jane Roe v. Henry Wade*, in which the Court held that the doctor had the absolute right, in his medical discretion, to take the life of a human fetus at any time before the first trimester. Kell convincingly claimed that the decision "created a hideous anomaly in the law," in that the cancer patient does not have the freedom of choice in preserving his own life that the mother has in taking the life of a fetus.

While the legal front kept Laetrile, or vitamin B-17, in the news, personalities also played a key role. It was at a Los Angeles convention of the Cancer Control Society in the summer of 1973 that Alycia Buttons, wife of comedian Red Buttons, announced that she had been rescued from death's door by amygdalin — a testimony she shared with several hundred other cancer patients meeting at a conference which would have been forbidden two years earlier.

Of equal impact at the convention was word from Laetrile's only "inside" battler, Dr. Dean Burk, head of the federally funded National Cancer Institute's cytochemistry division. Dr. Burk was a major gadfly in the side of the medical-bureaucratic establishment. He announced that Memorial Sloan-Kettering Cancer Center in New York had begun the serious testing of Laetrile, with the chairman of President Nixon's advisory board, which supervises the administration's National Cancer Plan, playing a direct role. The tests on mice were actually well under way, and as the advisory board chairman, investment banker Benno C. Schmidt, told the *Associated Press*, Sloan-Kettering began its studies after he had received "hundreds of letters about Laetrile and began to look into the matter." Finally, Laetrile was on the way to getting at least a partial hearing at one of the major cancer research institutions in the country.

For Dean Burk, a biochemist who had openly and vociferously assailed medical officialdom for years for its refusal to clear Laetrile for tests on humans, Sloan-Kettering's interest represented a major victory — a milestone on the road to possible legalization. His sentiments were echoed months later by Sloan-Kettering itself. In a preliminary report on Laetrile tests on mice, purposely leaked to the press (not by the institution itself) as an adjunct to the Richardson case, it was revealed that in a ten-month series of experiments involving a strain of mice that develop breast cancer, Laetrile doses caused "significant inhibition of the formation of lung metastases," and "possibly prevents, to an uncertain degree, the formation of new tumors. . . ." The impact of the news was traumatic.

For the first time, a prestigious and "orthodox" cancer facility in the United States had conducted controlled tests, however narrow of range, in a thorough, scientific way, and had come up with positive results. Even later Sloan-Kettering statements that another series of tests had failed to confirm the earlier results failed to dim the enthusiasm of the laetrilists. As Ernst Krebs, Jr. observed, there was no way to erase the results of the earlier tests.

The early release of positive test data embarassed Sloan-Kettering. A researcher on the project told me that he personally was disgruntled by the early "leak," and that it was too early to make sweeping generalizations. Yet he added he was moving toward the point of view that nutrition plays an overwhelming role in cancer prevention.

Perhaps the best reporting on the Sloan-Kettering matter was that in *Science* magazine by Barbara J. Culliton, who noted that "the conclusion Sloan-Kettering scientists draw from these [mice] data is that Laetrile is worth further study, even though there is no convincing scientific basis for its use in human beings as yet." She quoted Benno Schmidt: "Since I've been chairman of the President's cancer panel, I've had literally hundreds of letters about Laetrile. Some people ask me whether it is any good. Others flatly say that, in any case, it alleviates pain. When I answer these people and tell them that Laetrile has no effect, I would like to be able to do so with some conviction."

Taking the matter up with the National Cancer Institute — whose cytochemistry chief, Dean Burk, vigorously and outspokenly dissented from the NCI view — Schmidt was told that Laetrile had been looked into and that there was no basis for claims made about Laetrile's capability as a cancer fighter. He heard the same story from the American Cancer Society. But, he recalled, when he asked for evidence, "I couldn't get anybody to show me his work."[4]

Dr. Chester Stock, vice president of Sloan-Kettering, commented for *Associated Press* on the mixed results of the S-K tests. His investigators, he said, had not been able to show, under the conditions used, that there is the precise difference between cancer and normal cells (in suggested enzyme activity releasing cyanide at cancer sites) that Laetrile's defenders claim. "We think it's just flawed theory," he said. But that there could be other mechanisms at work that might produce an anticancer effect, he said, seemed obvious since two sets of Sugiura experiments showed that:

1. Larger tumors did not stop growing when amygdalin was used — but smaller tumors in general did not grow any further.

2. Results of metastases (spread) cancer were more interesting. Of the mice at the end of the experiment which were not treated, eighteen or 78.2 percent had lung metastases present. Of those treated with amygdalin, only four or 17.4 percent exhibited metastases.[5]

There then began an incredible saga at Sloan-Kettering — one not yet finished as this was written.

First, as the budding author of *Vitamin B-17: Forbidden Weapon Against Cancer*, I wanted to check the most recent rumors about a *third* test at Sloan-Kettering with officials there. I had heard that this third test tended to confirm the first, and that on the basis of this, the institute was planning human studies in conjunction with a hospital in Mexico City. I approached S-K officials with these reports in October 1974 and they confirmed both, which led to an enthusiastic preface to my first book.

As a journalist in hot pursuit of a fascinating story, and an observer of the rapidly growing Laetrile War, I sat back awaiting some kind of official announcement from Sloan-Kettering. It was a long wait.

In January 1975 a Sloan-Kettering vice president told Canadian national television that "we have seen results which seem to be significant" in Laetrile tests on mice. A few months later, another Sloan-Kettering officer was quoted as saying the Laetrile tests had shown the substance to be worthless. He later issued a statement in effect denying the printed remark and said that the tests were continuing.

In July 1975 S-K spokesmen told the *New York Times* that independent tests of Laetrile on mouse cancer systems had not been able to duplicate (or "replicate," as goes the scientific jargon) Dr. Sugiura's earlier work, that the earlier test had been "spurious," despite the fact that it had been carried out by Dr. Sugiura, one of the foremost researchers in the field. The officials said there was now simply no "scientific justification for testing Laetrile as a possbile therapy for cancer patients."

The *New York Times* statements, if they were intended to have a cooling effect on the matter, boomeranged:

Somebody at Sloan-Kettering sent me, on S-K letterhead, the following letter, marked as received August 23, 1975:

> *Dear Mr. Culbert:*
>
> *Here are some [sic] the results of Sloan-Kettering's experiments with Laetrile. Due to political pressure these results are being suppressed. Please do your best to bring these important finds to the attention of the people. Krebs' theory is very promising, and Laetrile should be tested to see if it really holds water.*

There was no signature. Attached were 32 pages, including tables, notes, and typed memoranda, of *six* sets of tests, all carried out by Dr. Sugiura, between August 3, 1973, and February 8, 1975, *all* of which showed positive effects from Laetrile on specific mouse cancers, particularly in the blocking of the spread (or "metastasis") of cancer. Here indeed was a bombshell — it showed that in *seven* sets of tests Laetrile had demonstrated positive anti-cancer effects! I instantly moved to confirm the authenticity of the reports. It was confirmed by S-K itself that the reports were genuine, and it was also made clear that Dr. Sugiura had *not* sent me the note.

Because of the cavalier put-down of Laetrile by Sloan-Kettering, through the *New York Times*, and the subsequent coverup, and the feeling by the Committee for Freedom of Choice that the first "leaked" report would probably never have seen the light of day had it not been leaked, the Committee published all sets of Sugiura's studies in a small volume entitled *Anatomy of a Coverup*.

In it, Dr. Ernst T. Krebs, Jr. appropriately summarized:

> *Those who recognize as overwhelmingly important and decisive the criterion of the total inhibition of such metastases from a primary tumefaction see in Sugiura's findings a 70-percent total inhibition of such metastases in Laetrile-treated mice, as compared to controls, an experiment that at present not only proves the anti-neoplastic action of Laetrile, but proves it with a total success rate of at least 70 percent.[6]*

If it had been embarrassed before by the single "leak," Sloan-Kettering was now triply miffed at the six-way deluge.

After both the Committee and IACVF announced the "coverup" in meetings in the United States and Canada in September, Sloan-Kettering enlisted the pages of *Medical World News*[7] to deny the coverup.

In what *MWN* called an unprecedented action for the research institute, S-K spokesmen went on record to claim that:

The Committee had "purloined" *selective* test data which were "out of date" and that the following negative Laetrile-mice tests had been conducted: two by Surgeon Daniel S. Martin, Catholic Medical Center, Queens, N.Y., mid-1974; two by immunologist Elizabeth S. Stockert in 1975; and two more by research veterinarian Franz A. Schmid, Dr. Sugiura's son-in-law. *MWN* did quote Sugiura as saying: "It is still my belief that amygdalin cures metastases."

Significantly, however, S-K spokesmen made no effort to deny the authenticity of the seven sets of Sugiura data. Of course the Committee had purloined nothing. Too, test data as late as 1975 could hardly be said to be "out of date." But most important, in the specific variety of tumor system Sugiura was studying, never had any agent before Laetrile been found to exert a positive effect.

Since S-K spokesmen had denied that human tests had ever been planned — while the Committee reproduced correspondence between S-K and a Mexican hospital proving that such tests *had* been planned — the New York institute spokesmen explained that proposed collaborative trials were dropped "when negative evidence began to emerge in 1974 and 1975." This was at least a public admission that the trials had, in fact, been projected.

Sloan-Kettering announced that Drs. Sugiura and Schmid would undertake a joint series of tests in order to help clarify the issue one way or another — although to laetrilists the issue was already clarified: a "shred of evidence" from Laetrile use on mouse cancer had been achieved, and there was no way to wish away the results or to rewrite history.

Luckily, Hearst newspaper reporter Mort Young had begun the most thorough, objective, in-depth look at the whole issue ever undertaken by major media. In November, he reported that "early results" of the Sugiura-Schmid tests on mice highly susceptible to lung cancer broke down this way:

In the Sugiura test, 75 percent of "control" mice developed metastases against 23 percent of those treated with Laetrile. In the Schmid test, 100 percent of "control" mice had metastases against 31 percent of those treated with Laetrile. Young wrote: "These tests represent the first instance that Dr. Schmid's results come close to those of Dr. Sugiura. It is a dramatic reversal of Dr. Schmid's previous tests."

But by now S-K officialdom was maintaining a hermetic silence about what was going on. Dr. Sugiura continued to stand by his results, both in telephone chats I had with him as late as June 1976 and in written notes to medical students. A major Sloan-Kettering official told me in

June 1976 that the early but incomplete Schmid results were, indeed, "tending to confirm" the Sugiura ones, but that nothing decisive could be said until the fall of 1976.

In the meantime, David M. Rorvik, a scientifically oriented freelance writer working on a grant from the Alicia Patterson Foundation and specializing in politics and cancer research, also probed the ongoing Sloan-Kettering controversy. He found, among many other things, that even in Dr. Schmid's original negative results amygdalin-treated mice were living longer, even *with* lung cancer metastases — at ratios of 30 and 55 percent longer. Rorvik commented:

> *The [mouse] survival times were not emphasized, I was told, because the design of the test was to assess metastases. But, surely, to overlook a promising effect which arises, however serendipitously or incidentally in the course of studying another effect, cannot be characterized as good science. This effect should have been isolated and followed up — particularly since the anecdotal clinical evidence suggests that human cancer victims using Laetrile often survive in relative good health far beyond what the statistics say should be expected despite the presence and even continued spread of metastases. To the cancer victim, life — not metastases — is what it's all about.*[8]

In the Sugiura-Schmid cooperative study, Rorvik notes in the same report, "when I asked for the figures I was dumbfounded to learn that, depending upon which way one questionable mouse was 'analyzed,' either 73 percent of the controls and 44 percent of the Laetrile-treated animals had lung metastases or 80 percent of the controls and 44 percent of the treated animals had metastases. This was not statistically significant?"

He also quoted one official when challenged about his statements on consistently negative Laetrile results at S-K: "I say we have had negative results but I guess I should put it another way and say we haven't had consistently positive results and we don't feel we have something unless we do have."

Dr. Lloyd J. Old, an S-K vice president and associate director, had earlier uttered what probably was the most significant statement in the entire Sloan-Kettering controversy: "It may not be possible to ask the mouse for a final answer in this area."

Of *course* not.

"There are obviously tremendous differences between metabolisms of human and mouse [tumor] cells," cancer experts themselves have noted.[9]

Whether Laetrile tests on mice were all positive or negative, they could not possibly answer the only question that matters:

Is Laetrile effective in *man?*

But the overwhelming importance of the S-K controversy, its mixed results, and its contradictions, is this:

Even submitting Laetrile to detailed animal studies as a "cancer drug," Laetrile did *not* flunk. The only adequate model for total metabolic therapy with vitamin B-17 in human cancer is, of course, *man.* Yet, as we will see, even domesticated animals are responding to vitamin B-17 therapy.

The Sloan-Kettering results, either partly positive or wholly positive, depending on the criteria one is using (are we measuring tumor reduction, life-extension or feeling of well-being or all of these?), now provide important data that Laetrile *has* "checked out" in animal studies. But the Sloan-Kettering results are not the only examples available.

While the partially successful results at Sloan-Kettering were fresh in mind, more news was forthcoming at an international meeting in Baden-Baden, West Germany. Results of successful treatment of mouse tumors with amygdalin had come from the Manfred von Ardenne Research Institute in Dresden. A translation of the report, "Prolongation of Life in Tumor-Bearing Mice by Bitter Almonds," summarized: "In mice with Ehrlich ascites carcinoma, bitter almonds taken in addition to standard feed in a free food choice caused a significant prolongation of survival time, which is associated with inhibition of tumor growth."[10]

The Dresden report was crucial: bitter almonds are a primary source of the specific chemical substance (beta-cyanogenetic glucosides — or "nitriloside," as coined by biochemist Ernst T. Krebs, Jr.) that the laetrilists assert is both a preventative against cancer and a "control" for it.

Back in the United States, however, the official position remained inflexibly the same — and the National Cancer Institute pointed to a whole new set of statistics to justify it. On December 19, 1973, Saul A. Schepartz, associate director for drug research and development at the institute, released this statement:

> *I am attaching a report from Southern Research Institute summarizing and evaluating four experiments that we carried out with Amygdalin MF against the Lewis lung carcinoma. Based on this total experience, the conclusion has been reached that this material does not possess activity in the Lewis lung carcinoma system. We had previously reported that Amygdalin MF had been tested in a variety of other experimental tumor systems without evidence of activity. With the receipt of this report, we have now completed all of our projected testing with Amygdalin MF. Based on all of the studies we have carried out, we conclude that the material does not possess activity in any of the tumor*

systems that we have utilized. No further experiments are contemplated at this time.[11]

This kind of summary further bolstered the NCI's official position, as stated by C. Gordon Zubrod, director of the institute's Division of Cancer Treatment: "Laetrile (Amygdalin MF) is not considered a recognized treatment for cancer. Although Laetrile has been widely used in a number of countries, claims concerning its effectiveness are based on anecdotal reports and to our knowledge the type of carefully controlled clinical study necessary to determine the properties of an anticancer drug has been neither conducted abroad nor reported."[12] The Zubrod statement recalled earlier NCI tests that had been dismissed as negative.

To all of which Dr. Dean Burk said, "Nonsense!" — as he had statistically demonstrated on prior occasions, in which he dissented from the global conclusions reached by the NCI at the end of its studies. Burk declared in February 1974 that the Southern Research Institute studies make a case for the efficacy of Laetrile rather than its worthlessness. "You may say the evidence is not only overwhelming — it is overwhelmingly overwhelming," the veteran scientist told me. This was the same outspoken researcher who frequently referred to the "output of obfuscations, deceptions, deviousness, red herrings, or actual lies regarding Laetrile," and who observed in a letter to a congressman: "Once any of the FDA NCI-AMA-ACS hierarchy so much as concedes that Laetrile antitumor efficacy was indeed even once observed in NCI experimentation, a permanent crack in the bureaucratic armor has taken place that can widen indefinitely by further appropriate experimentation." Burk's counter-studies are at least evidence that experts can disagree on findings.

I should once again strongly reiterate that neither Dr. Burk, nor Laetrile's developer and pioneer, Ernst T. Krebs, Jr. nor the Laetrile-using physicians around the world have ever regarded vitamin B-17 as a *cure* for cancer. In its oral and injectable form, they insist it is the best cancer weapon we have. The most exciting possibility of all, of course, is their insistence that vitamin B-17 may be *the* preventative against cancer; that if enough of the vitamin were taken through natural foods, there would not be any need for the processed, commercial product called Laetrile.

As a newspaperman, I covered the vitamin B-17 story in starts and stops since 1971. I interviewed a score of people in the Bay Area who told of seemingly incredible "controls" accomplished through cancer therapy centered on vitamin B-17. At the Richardson trials scores of new testimonials were given to me by members of the Committee for Freedom of Choice in Cancer Therapy who were patients of Richardson, Contreras, or Hans Nieper. From what my interviewees told me — all in such glaring contradiction with what officialdom told me — it seemed from the outset that there was more to Laetrile than the bureaucratic dismissals of it would indicate.

I interviewed Dr. Ernesto Contreras in Tijuana, Dr. Dean Burk during his trips to the West Coast, and biochemist Ernst T. Krebs, Jr., frequently and exhaustively. I met with Dr. Manuel Navarro in the Philippines for his views, with Dr. Stewart Jones in Palo Alto, California, and was in touch with other researchers and with case histories and medical reports. As I crisscrossed the nation and visited other countries from 1974 through 1976, in a continuing investigation of vitamin B-17, I came across increasing numbers of testimonials — life-and-death battles of cancer patients which the FDA haughtily dismissed as "anectodal evidence." I met more and more doctors who were turning to the use of Laetrile as they saw their patients treated in the "orthodox" way dropping like flies. Doctors by the hundreds expressed more and more interest in Laetrile and its allied therapy and, while sneered at by their local medical associations, openly sought such information.

Fascinating questions nagged: Is it possible that cancer, in its cause, treatment, and prevention, involves a simple answer? If the substance vitamin B-17 is legal for use elsewhere, why the almost frantic rejection of it in the United States? Are thousands of Laetrile users and a substantial number of scientific supporters of the Krebs theory and product all deluded? As a layman, I cannot now say I have all the answers. But I have vigorously pursued the questions.

Several patterns have emerged in this investigation:

First, there obviously have been benefits, ranging from minimal to substantial, in Laetrile therapy. But best results are *not* obtained simply by injecting the substance or giving tablets. The *best* results are achieved when a full program of nutritional or metabolic therapy is involved; this includes a major dietary change and the use of other vitamins, enzymes and minerals.

The chemistry of "how Laetrile works" remains an open question. The local, cyanide-benzaldehyde-release theory of Dr. Krebs may be the answer in many cases, but the surveillant action of B-17 probably has a range of other chemical involvements. Dr. Krebs is no egotist; he does not take author's pride in the single-action theory of amygdalin. "It takes one explorer to discover the North Pole, another to map it," he told me in examining other theories as to the way in which the substance "works."

Scattered evidence exists that natural vitamin B-17 in sufficient quantity is as therapeutically good, if not better, than Laetrile itself, although not enough information has accrued for any substantive statements. Natural vitamin B-17 (the nitrilosides themselves in an abundant number of fruits, vegetables, seeds and grasses), in conjunction with other enzymes and involved in chemical actions not yet clear to researchers, may explain such dramatic cancer reversals as those obtained in Indonesia with the cuttings of cassava. And it may be that there are other substances in plant material complementary to, and as important as, vitamin B-17, which also exert a surveillant or therapeutic action against cancer.

Evidence of profound importance was developing from California veterinarians that domesticated dogs and cats — subjected to the same unnatural diets as their masters — were responding to vitamin B-17, either in Laetrile form or simply through the addition of apricot kernels to their food.

Most important, the dietary universe in which vitamin B-17 plays so strong a galactic role *seems* to be the key to longevity, good health, and the control or even defeat of degenerative disease. The dietary evidence from such disparate peoples as the Arctic Circle Eskimos (those uncontaminated by modern diet), the Abkhasians of the Soviet Union, the Vilcabamba Indians of Ecuador, the Hunzakuts of Pakistan (those remaining in their valley), certain Nigerian tribes, the rural Filipinos (those who have not migrated to the major cities or otherwise profoundly altered their high nitrilosidic and low-animal protein diets), certain American Indian groups, and many rural peoples of Asia, let alone the statistical evidence from such "civilized" groups as Seventh-Day Adventists in California and the Mormon-dominated populace of Utah, suggests longer life, better health, and less degenerative disease from a more-vegetarian, more-natural food, lower-animal protein, lower-fat diet.

CHAPTER THREE

From Death's Door:
The Laetrile Recoveries

KANSAS SALESMAN GLEN RUTHERFORD was told in 1971 that he had invasive adenocarcinoma of the lower intestine — cancer — that he should undergo surgery at once, and that removal of the rectum might be necessary.

Instead, the independent-minded Rutherford, hearing of the "Tijuana connection," went to Dr. Ernesto Contreras' Centro Medico Del Mar clinic for examination and treatment. He received Laetrile for several weeks under the supervision of Dr. Carlos Lopez — and his cancer symptoms disappeared.

The Rutherford case was precedent-setting for several reasons:

First, his diagnosis had been made in the United States by respected "orthodox" physicians.

Second, his treatment consisted only of Vitamin B-17 (Laetrile) and related therapy (radical change of diet, use of other vitamins and enzymes). That is to say, he had *not* undergone surgery, chemotherapy or radiation, so his total remission of symptoms could not be ascribed to a tardy reaction to orthodox treatment. *Medical World News* for June 28, 1976, somewhat sneeringly sought to suggest that since the malignant growth had indeed been cauterized — though *after* it had, in Rutherford's words, "shrunk from the size of an orange to that of a grape" — that the cauterization itself was the "cure." But Rutherford's chronic rectal bleeding, which first began in 1969, stopped after *five days* of 3-gram intravenous Laetrile injections daily and *something* shrank the malignancy.

Third, adequate followup confirmed his control of cancer. By 1976, he had completed five years without symptoms and — under the guidelines of medical orthodoxy — could be described as "cured." But he religiously stayed on maintenance levels of Vitamin B-17, other vitamins and enzymes.

Most important, he became the chief surviving member in a class action suit instituted in 1975 before the Western Oklahoma United States District Court. Under the terms of the suit, the Food and Drug Administration was enjoined from interfering with the right of Rutherford and a class of citizens — cancer patients defined as "terminal" — to have access to Laetrile and/or anything else necessary for their continued existence.

By the time of the suit, Rutherford, who became an ardent spokesman for Laetrile, told me he needed $14 worth of Laetrile, vitamins and enzymes daily simply to stay alive. The suit filed by the late attorney Clyde Watts on behalf of Rutherford and the terminal cancer patients read, in part:

> The Court is compelled to find from the testimony and the exhibits that plaintiff Glen L. Rutherford was in late 1971 suffering from invasive carcinoma, and that by the use of Laetrile, B-17 or amygdalin (all being the same drug) his condition was cured, as there is no evidence to the contrary.

> The Court finds that the plaintiff Rutherford is not free to have shipped to him, nor is he free to directly purchase and bring back to the United States from Mexico quantities of Laetrile for preventative treatment of his cancer. To do so would violate the law and would subject him to criminal prosecution. . . .

> In this connection the Court finds that Laetrile has been in use for a number of years in Mexico and other nations around the world, that the FDA has by its regulations made it impossible for the common man to have an application processed through FDA so that said agency would either approve or disapprove the drug known as Laetrile.

> The Court finds that Congress intended by 21 U.S.C. Section 355 that the FDA would on its own initiative approve or disapprove the use of Laetrile as a freedom of choice by those suffering from cancer to use in lieu of surgery or radiation cobalt treatment.

> The Court finds that the FDA has abdicated its duty to make a clear determination of whether the drug Laetrile should or should not be placed in commerce though the drug has been in use for many years and thousands of persons have been treated with it.

> The Court finds from the record, testimony and exhibits that Laetrile is not lethal in any sense of the word. It is not harmful to the human body and when used in proper amounts under proper control and supervision can effect relief from cancer disease to the satisfaction of many who are privileged to use the same.

The Court further finds from the record that the plaintiff Ruther-ford herein and those similarly situated have been denied this right of choice in using B-17 or Laetrile without just cause on the part of the Secretary of HEW and its agency FDA.

Inaction by the FDA constitutes the crux of plaintiff's procedural dilemma, and the question arises relevant to plaintiff's request for equitable relief, as to whether an interpretation or construction of Section 355 authorizes such inaction and is in keeping with the Congressional intent the statute embodies . . . .

It can be seen that the statute allows but two alternatives: the issuance of an order approving the application or the issuance of an order refusing to approve the application. The evidence does not reflect the Secretary to have done either . . . .

Thus the statutory duty has not been carried out and cancer victims have thereby been placed in limbo with regard to Laetrile, unable to invoke the jurisdiction of the courts. Since the Secretary has failed to act, the Court must act on behalf of this plaintiff who has been adversely affected by such failure. Congress has not legislated a statute which can be used by silence and inaction to still the clamor and demands of citizens, especially those nearly 1,000 who die each day of cancer . . . .

The Court finds from the evidence that Laetrile is not a toxic or harmful substance if used in proper dosage but is on the other hand an alternative treatment of cancer which can be used in lieu of surgery or radiation cobalt.

Rutherford's case was only one of many which began surfacing in 1975 and which conflicted with the "establishment" explanation of Laetrile effectiveness: namely, that persons with seeming recoveries from Laetrile therapy fell into one or more of the following categories:

(a) They had never had cancer in the first place and/or they had been improperly diagnosed; (b) they were responding tardily to earlier orthodox treatment; (c) they had undergone "spontaneous remission" — a phrase the "counter-culture" of the 1960s and 1970s correctly refers to as a "cop-out," a way for orthodoxy to say in effect that "something just happened — we don't know why, but it certainly couldn't have anything to do with that quack remedy."

Rutherford's case met the criterion of the defenders of orthodoxy when they insisted: "Show us the records."

Even so, orthodoxy could fall back on the mystery of cancer itself: *some* cancers do, indeed, seem spontaneously to disappear, or to "undergo remission." Laetrile adherents do not duck this fact — they simply challenge orthodoxy to compare the numbers of "spontaneous remissions" of Laetrile patients with the number of "spontaneous remissions" of patients on, say, such orthodox chemotherapies as 5-Fu or cyclophosphamide.

By 1975 and 1976 an increasing number of cancer-control cases were coming from persons who had been diagnosed and treated with Laetrile therapy only *inside* the United States — no small part of such cases being directly due to the organizing efforts of the Committee for Freedom of Choice in Cancer Therapy, Inc., which claimed a leap in "medical arts" membership of from 5 to 1100 in four years' time. This number included more than 50 doctors who were openly using Laetrile in their medical practice.

Wherever the Committee went, organizing more than 400 chapters across the country, it learned of spectacular new cases demonstrating vitamin B-17 effectiveness.

For example, in Greensboro, N.C., a 21-year-old student made the case for Laetrile better than any Committee spokesman could. Pam McDaniel of High Point shared her testimonial on television; she was interviewed by the Committee publication *The Choice* in its June 1976 issue:

> She was diagnosed in March 1975 with terminal, metastasized osteosarcoma (bone cancer in both legs spread to other parts of the body), and, "I was told not to expect to see Christmas 1975. I was using crutches, my legs were locking. The doctors were honest enough to tell me it would be useless to try chemotherapy, and they also said radiation would burn everything before it even got to the leg bones." She was also in great pain.
>
> Ultimately, Pam McDaniel saw 21 doctors before four concurred in her diagnosis. The best they could offer her, she said, was surgery, or the lopping off of both legs. Even with that, they warned, there would still be a 50-50 chance she would be paralyzed from the hips down.
>
> She was told to go home and make out a will. Deeply religious, Pam McDaniel took her problem to God.
>
> She finally learned about Laetrile (vitamin B-17) and was able to make connections with a doctor in the South — one who subsequently went under fire from his state medical board for daring to use Laetrile in cancer therapy.
>
> The important element in this case is that Miss McDaniel eventually took the Laetrile therapy only — no surgery, no chemotherapy, no

radiation. She received 20 cc of Laetrile intravenously every day for 43 days, then 20cc every three days, and then one injection and one tablet every other day.

Her former doctors were amazed that as of spring 1976 she was without a trace of cancer.

While it was too early to make long-term claims for such a dramatic case, Miss McDaniel had already received obvious visible benefits from going the way of "unorthodoxy." Since hers was a documented case of U.S.-diagnosed, U.S.-treated, Laetrile-only therapy, the only "excuse" for her complete turnaround in the view of orthodoxy would have to be "spontaneous remission."

Among well-documented, U.S.-treatment-only cases the Committee came across, which were subsequently reported in *The Choice*, were the stories of Harold Barber and Pat Smith:

Barber, a retired engineer from Hattiesburg, Miss., was diagnosed in 1969 with cancer of the bladder. Between January 1969 and October 1973 he underwent three operations on the bladder, each taking away more of the organ until after the last surgery more than seven-eighths of his bladder had been removed.

In February 1974, he went to see a Laetrile-using physician in Georgia who put him on 9 grams of intravenous Laetrile (vitamin B-17) every other day, or a total of 11 treatments, plus 150-mg. B-17 tablets every other day, special enzymes and other vitamins. His diet was also changed to the low-animal protein, mostly-vegetarian regimen suggested for cancer cases.

Following this, Barber told The Choice *in April 1976, he went on and off the vials and tablets until August 1975, when a recurrence was noted and tumor was observed blocking the kidneys. At death's door due to uremia, Barber was placed on a dialysis machine and sent to M.D. Anderson Hospital in Dallas for chemotherapy since doctors now termed his recurred bladder cancer inoperable. He said that "doctors later told me I was written off as dead in August." He was scheduled to take 12 chemotherapy treatments, but could only stand four since "I lost 20 pounds, all of my hair, and could hardly walk across the room. I refused to take more chemotherapy."*

Barber then went back to Laetrile therapy, taking 9 grams intravenously and daily for 20 days, and then cutting back to 6 grams per week along with two 500-mg. tablets five days per week. He began treating himself and as of March 1976 he was x-rayed "A to Z" in Hattiesburg.

"There was no evidence of cancer — and the records are on file," he asserted. Barber said some of his earlier physicians claimed his total absence of cancer was a "delayed reaction" to the four shots of chemotherapeutic agents.

Pat Smith, a 54-year-old real estate broker from Columbia, South Carolina, told the committee of his well-documented total control of metastasized stomach cancer with Laetrile (vitamin B-17) and the ancillary diet.

Diagnosed in May 1975, Smith at the time had such an enormous abdominal extension, due to stomach acid and pleural discharge, that at one time he was inflated with two gallons — 25 lbs. — of such fluid.

Diagnosed and treated in the South, he started out in June 1975 on daily 3-gram vials of intravenous Laetrile, along with Vitamins C and E, special enzymes, and six tablets of Vitamin B-15 daily. He later switched to two 20-cc injections of Laetrile per week along with three 500-mg tablets of B-17 per week.

His prior doctors had warned him that chemotherapy is poison, so he had abstained from trying that "orthodox" route. He also turned down surgery.

The result, as of April 1976, when he met with Committee spokesmen in Columbia, S.C., was total control of cancer. X-rays had confirmed both the absence of tumors and the complete disappearance of stomach liquid.

"I would have died last August or September without it," he said of the Laetrile-dietary treatment.

Again, it was too early in the usual five-year span of survival time to talk about either total control or cure, but the results plainly show dramatic effects from the Laetrile program, whether those effects turn out to be temporary or enduring.

A 48-year-old insurance salesman from Baton Rouge, Louisiana, also provided *The Choice* with well-documented information on cancer control through Laetrile (Vitamin B-17) therapy:

Billy Williams was given two to six weeks to live in 1975 following diagnosis of, and surgery for, lung cancer.

In January 1975, Mr. Williams, of Baton Rouge, La., complained of loss of energy and was consistently tired, symptoms which continued for months. He entered a Baton Rouge hospital May 12 — for surgery following a ruptured hernia. Many x-rays were taken at the time and he still did not feel "right" after the operation. His weight had already dropped from 240 to 195 lbs., by the time he returned to the hospital at the end of June. Following an esophagoscopy, diagnosis of lung cancer was made.

Surgery was performed on July 10, but Williams was warned at the time that the surgeons had not "gotten it all" and advised him to go the radiation and chemotherapy route.

"I had seen the results of radiation and chemotherapy on other people — that's why I chose Laetrile," he told The Choice.

Down to 175 lbs., Williams sought out a B-17-using physician in Birmingham, Ala., starting July 24, 1975. He was placed on a schedule of three 3-gram Laetrile vials every other day for a total of 48 vials and 500-mg. tablets on the other days. He was also given Viokase and Ananase enzymes, Vitamins C, E and B-15, Theragran-M, minerals, various B vitamins and orotates, brewer's yeast and acidophilus, and was placed on a detoxification program. His cancer metastasis disappeared.

Blood tests and x-rays were taken August 2 and August 25. He was responding though his weight reached a low of 165 lbs. He became a patient of Dr. S. R. "Pete" Abramson in Marksville, La., August 25, and started a 15-day program of 3 vials daily and 19 weeks of single 500-mg. tablets six days a week, followed by 5-cc injections in each hip on the set th *day for 19 weeks.*

By January 22, 1976, his weight had climbed to 214 lbs. and a Baton Rouge doctor found that there is "no evidence of an active process in the lungs . . . no evidence of tumor."

Despite being told following lung surgery and his refusal to try radiation and chemotherapy that he might have only two to six weeks to live, Williams had survived for a year by the time I talked to him in May, 1976, was restored to health, and was taking a single 500-mg. B-17 tablet daily along with enzymes, vitamins and minerals.

Checkups in April and May showed him to be cancer-free.

Williams' case was particularly compelling since he had been diagnosed and treated only in the United States and exclusively with Laetrile and its ancillary therapy. Moreover, he had the documents to prove his response.

During the 1976 indictments against the Laetrile "smugglers" and the press attacks on the Mexican clinics and Laetrile doctors as engaging in a "ripoff of desperate cancer patients," the case of Charles W. Sittig of Irving, Texas, was also made known to *The Choice*. Telling Sittig that the Contreras Clinic was a "ripoff" was enough to bring the Texan to a boil:

For Sittig, a 54-year-old salesman who was diagnosed with melanoma in June 1975 and who decided to go the Vitamin B-17 route in Tijuana, instead, believes his treatment there saved his life and stopped

*the melanoma — and did so at a cost far under what he would have paid
in this country.*

His story:

*Diagnosed in a Texas hospital on June 5 with melanoma on the
right calf, Sittig underwent an operation, but the knife did not "get it
all." During a checkup on December 15, 1975, a swelling in the groin
was found and massive groin surgery for the metastasized cancer was
suggested.*

*Sittig refused the idea of a second surgery and also turned down the
idea he should be used to experiment with BCG treatment, then touted as
a new "breakthrough" in cancer. "I found out it might have killed me,"
he told* The Choice.

*Instead, the Texan, feeling fatigued, limping and agonizing over
swollen hands, went to the Del Mar Clinic of Dr. Ernesto Contreras in
Tijuana for a three-week assault on his cancer problem.*

*But the going wasn't all that easy. "I literally had to fight (the
original hospital) just to get my pathology report and other records. I
finally got them when I said I was going to Houston for treatment," he
said. Among the reports, intriguingly enough, is the contradiction in his
diagnosis: one report referred to his cancer as not being "vascular
invasive"; another claimed it was "definitely invasive."*

*In Tijuana, Sittig went through a detoxification program, went on
the Laetrile diet, rectal enzymes and one 3-gram vial of intravenous
Laetrile daily six days a week for three weeks.*

*"A few days later my limp disappeared, and I noticed I could get
my ring off my finger again. Even boils on my back disappeared."*

*Apparently without any sign of cancer, Sittig was referred to the
Ft. Worth Medical Center for a "scan" to see just how complete his
recovery was. Sittig remembers the cost involved with some chagrin:*

*"For $7 I had a checkup at the Contreras clinic to pronounce me
free of cancer. But in Texas all this checking cost $800 — to say nothing
of the $50 office call and the $50 so-called 'room entry' fee." He was
found to be cancer-free.*

*"All my expenses in Tijuana came to around $2,000, including six
months of medicine to take home. The treatment cost $11 a day there,"
he said.*

Equal praise for Contreras came from literally thousands of his
patients. The case of Ft. Pierce, Florida insurance agent James W.
Sowinski might be considered typical. In a testimonial (in *The Choice* for
March, 1976) dated October 18, 1975, Sowinski gave this account:

"In November, 1972, I was stricken with hypernephroma, a

cancer of the left kidney. Upon seeing urologists in West Palm Beach, Fla., it was decided due to the size of the tumor to treat me with x-ray radiation prior to surgery in order to try to shrink the size of the tumor and thereby make it more operable.

"Surgery was performed at Good Samaritan Hospital in West Palm Beach December 11, 1972. I was on the operating table for 6½ hours and was told I died twice on the operating table. There was heavy bleeding during surgery and I received a total of 19 pints of blood, 17 during surgery and two after surgery. Due to the heavy bleeding the doctors were unable to remove the entire tumor, leaving a portion about the size of an egg above the kidney area. Of course my left kidney was removed as it was completely destroyed by the cancer. The cancer had spread from the primary area up into the muscle system above the kidney. My surgeon said that the most likely area for the cancer to move to then was the lungs.

"The radiologist suggested another series of X-ray radiation treatments to try to kill the remainder of the tumor which was left in me although he offered only about a 10% chance that it would help. My family was told that I had a very short time to live.

"Needless to say, many prayers were offered by myself, family and friends and I feel it is by the help of prayer that I am alive today. A lady from our church brought my wife information about Laetrile and her sister who had been cured of throat cancer by using Laetrile.

"After the second series of X-ray radiation treatments I told my doctor that I was going to Tijuana, Mexico, for Laetrile by Dr. Ernesto Contreras, M.D. He tried to discourage me but I told him I was going anyway. I started my Laetrile treatments the last Monday of February in 1973 and lasted for three weeks. After completing Laetrile injections in Mexico I returned home and have been taking the 500 mg Laetrile tablets. I returned to work April 1, 1973, and have been working a full schedule selling life insurance which calls for night work and long hours. I put in many 16-hour days at work. I am perfectly healthy now and feel better than I have in years. I will be 56 my next birthday in February.

"I would like to conclude by saying 'I Praise the Lord' for Laetrile and Dr. Contreras."

Mrs. O. C. (Betty) Elder of Birmingham, Alabama became virtually a one-woman voice for Laetrile (vitamin B-17) therapy in the South since her own amazing recovery from terminal cancer.

Deeply religious, Mrs. Elder told me she believes she was singled out to suffer the tragedy of cancer and permitted to see others suffering from it as well, so that she would "discover" Laetrile and help inform others about it. Her case is as dramatic as it is inspiring:

"*Before I was diagnosed with cancer, I was extremely tired,*" she said. "*Then I noticed a knot in my left armpit, which got very large. Then there was a small one under the right arm. They removed the large one (in 1970) and found it to be malignant. I then praised the Lord for it and I gave the Lord credit for everything. But God took this and used it in a beautiful way.*

"*The surgeon said I would be sent to the greatest cancer specialist (in Birmingham) to be treated for reticular cell sarcoma (lymph gland cancer). The specialist said he would give me chemotherapy. I asked what it did and he said, 'it won't cure you and it might kill you.' But he and the other doctors said they had to do something. He gave me four poisons in the bloodstream. Every day on this treatment I went home and spent six hours in the bathroom throwing up. Only then would the nausea leave.*

"*He then gave me Vincristine (following the other four toxic chemotherapies), and my hair began to fall out — probably as a response to all four poisons. My color began to change. I went through five months of that treatment — I was supposed to go for six, but I quit. It affected my equilibrium, my thinking, my eyes, my speech. I became bald again, I couldn't even hold a pen to write with, and I could only walk by holding on to ramps. But I never gave up. I couldn't sleep, and I just fought to live.*

"*A year passed. I had been off chemotherapy for that time, and a knot returned to my neck.*" She went back to the cancer specialist for two treatments of Vincristine as well as Prednisone hormone. "*This time my kidneys went bad. The cancer doctor was upset and told me he couldn't get enough cytotoxin in to have an effect. It's true that the knot went away, but my hair fell out again and I was in generally bad shape. In two months, another knot appeared. The surgeon said he couldn't keep on removing these knots as they were coming one after the other. Then I went back to the cancer specialist.*

"*At his clinic, I saw every kind of cancer — people in great pain, some with their faces eaten off, some with legs, breasts and arms removed, some bloated, some only skin and bones. God allowed me to go through this since I love Jesus and He had a job for me to do. I went back to the cancer doctor and he gave me a double dose of Vincristine (and two other modalities). Then my hair fell out for the third time. I was rushed to the hospital as an emergency case. That was 2½ years ago. I had fever, I was blistered inside, my teeth were loose, I had blisters in my nose. I stayed in the hospital and the surgeon pulled me through.*

"*I went back to the specialist and he said the chemotherapy wasn't working — not that it ever had. My blood count was down to half, and he said, 'You have less than six months to live.' That was in 1973. He said he would give me cobalt if I wanted it. I refused. I was sent in for a lymphangiogram. I walked down the hall with a hospital employee, an x-ray technician, who said he wanted to pray with me. His prayer was, 'Satan, I demand you in the name of Jesus, that you get out of this body because it belongs to Jesus.' He prayed to Jesus to heal my body.*

"*In the waiting room I saw patients being wheeled in. I began praying, asking for God to send a cure for everyone. I called up my prayer partners for them to ask God to send a cure.*"

Then a series of events occurred, she recalled. A cousin telephoned her to tell her about an Alabama physician who was using Laetrile in his practice. She talked to the doctor by telephone but still wasn't convinced. Then her nephew took the family cat to veterinarian Dr. Allen Price, Birmingham, for a checkup. While there, the nephew spotted a pamphlet Dr. Price had on the table — an article on Laetrile by Alan Stang. Dr. Price sent her back the article through her nephew.

"*I read it,*" *Mrs. Elder recalls.* "*I said, 'This is the answer.' I went to the Laetrile doctor, who ordered the medicine from Tennessee. I hobbled into his office in Vestalia for the first shot of nine grams.*" *She began receiving 9-gram injections every other day for a month and taking 10 100-mg Vitamin B-17 tablets daily along with three B-15 tablets, 1500 mg. of Vitamin C, 800 IU of Vitamin E, special enzymes and a multiple vitamin tablet. Her diet was also changed to remove all animal protein except for eggs. She cut down on sugar and coffee, gave up white bread and "ate everything raw I could find, and then chopped it up as a big salad" including onion and garlic.*

She followed this regimen for a month, and began feeling better than she had felt for years. When she returned to the Alabama cancer specialist, "he asked me if I was taking his medicine. I told him I was taking vitamins instead. He said there was nothing to it. But he also found that I had no cancer, and that I was feeling like a million. He went into a rage and left the room. Since that day I have had no cancer, and it's been about 30 months — and I feel wonderful."

Unfortunately, the doctor who treated her with Laetrile was under investigation by the Alabama state medical board and was forced to stop using Laetrile or lose his license.

Mrs. Elder is on the telephone daily to patients from throughout the country spreading the news about Laetrile.

"*I believe God is behind this,*" *she told me.*

It was on July 27, 1972, that the *Berkeley Daily Gazette* broke the story that a fifty-five-year-old "terminal cancer" patient from Pinole,

California, being operated on to reverse a colostomy, was discovered to have no sign of the dread disease at all.

The case of Dave Edmunds, a restaurateur was intriguing to this newsman, then beginning a probe of Laetrile, for these reasons: The diagnosis of his cancer had been made in the United States by American doctors; his treatment had continued in the United States; and the cancer-free diagnosis was also made in this country. The medication that Edmunds had been taking every day from December 1971 — after refusing cobalt — was Laetrile.

The way in which he secured the Laetrile and how it was administered to him had to remain a secret; after all, a well-known Bay Area hospital was involved and well-credentialed doctors had treated him, even though the hospital and his operating surgeons were "innocent" of having had anything to do with his Laetrile treatment.

The amazing case of Edmunds began late in 1969, when he noticed that his weight dropped thirty pounds in two months. Two doctors gave him injections and pills, and a third ordered him to a hospital for tests, which revealed an intestinal tumor. Told he would die without surgery, the individualistic Edmunds turned to his own attempt at control through fruit juices. His weight went from 160 to 112 pounds. He was hospitalized in June 1971 and a large section of his bowel was removed. He was left with a colostomy, or temporary artificial anus. Months later he was hospitalized again and a marble-sized tumor was removed from his bladder. It became apparent that the cancer tissue was still in his body. The surgeons said further surgery would do no good and they suggested cobalt.

Having read about Laetrile, and feeling desperate, Edmunds and his wife Josephine decided to turn — as, I later found, so many had turned — to Laetrile. He made contact through the "Laetrile underground" and began the treatment, beginning with three 3-gram injections every week and 1,500-milligram oral doses per day. By April 1972 injections were terminated and he continued only the daily doses of oral Laetrile. From the first use of Laetrile in December 1971, and through the time he was pronounced tumor-free, Edmunds insists he took no other treatment. He noted over the months that his general health began to improve — he gained weight, his appetite improved, his energy perked up, and he was suffering no side effects.

Before he was operated on for a third time, Edmunds stopped at a Richmond, California, hospital for an examination by the urologist. He recalls vividly the degree of excitement as the doctor, peering into his genitourinary areas in the uncomfortable way urologists do such things, could find no trace of malignancy. At another hospital, Edmunds was operated on by a doctor who said it would be a "waste of time" to reverse the colostomy if even a "trace" of cancer were found. No trace was found, and the operation occurred.

"They just don't understand it — they can't believe it, they think it's amazing," Edmunds elatedly told the *Gazette*. The Californian went on to become an outspoken defender of Laetrile, appearing in 1972 and 1973 at conferences and meetings as proof that an unorthodox approach to cancer had worked, at least in his case.

I later asked Edmunds on a television program if he thought during his unorthodox treatment that he had been "in the hands of kooks, cranks, and charlatans." He paused only momentarily before saying, "They were more like a band of angels."

Lorraine Clark, a Concord, California, housewife and an active Jehovah's Witness, was the first Laetrile patient I interviewed. Diagnosed and treated in Mexico, quite legally, by Dr. Ernesto Contreras, her case might well be pooh-poohed by those who distrust the Tijuana approach. But, like Edmunds later, Mrs. Clark was convinced she owed her life to the banned substance and she was always eager to say so.

She had first met Contreras when she took her father-in-law to see the Mexican medic. Frank Clark, also of Concord, was suffering from rectal cancer. Lorraine Clark had previously lost her parents and a brother to the disease, and now her father-in-law had been given three weeks to live by American doctors. Frank Clark underwent the Laetrile treatment and died eighteen months later, but not of cancer — he suffered a heart attack. During that time, Mrs. Clark swears, the Laetrile seemed to bring his cancer under control.

Mrs. Clark, originally told in October 1966 that she had a tumor in the uterine cervix, was examined in Tijuana. Dr. Contreras used the urine test for cancer — denounced by American medicine — and informed her that she should start taking Laetrile capsules. She continued taking the little yellow pills during 1967, finally attaining two "negative" readings. In June 1968 she returned to Tijuana, where Contreras judged her tumors now to be nonmalignant. She underwent a hysterectomy and a "quart of tumor" was removed.

She told me that the operation, regarded by her American doctors as "excellent," had buoyed up her spirits. Too much. Now overconfident, she believed the problem was over. She went off Laetrile, and was doing all right for months until she started having abdominal pains. A loss of eighteen pounds in two weeks told her all she needed to know. "It was my own fault," she said. Back in Tijuana in October 1969, she began "massive injections" of the substance. Since that time, she believes, her cancer has been "controlled." She was still healthy and "controlled" in January 1974.

The return of cancerous symptoms, she told me, was ample evidence for her of a key element in the Krebs theory — that Laetrile "controls" but does not "cure" cancer, as insulin controls but does not cure diabetes.

Why had she opted to take her father-in-law to Tijuana in the first place, I wanted to know. "I watched them cut my mother up piece by piece through three operations, a lot of misery and expense," she replied.

Mrs. Clark was vehement in her denunciations of the American Medical Association, the FDA, and everyone else involved in making the proffering of Laetrile for cancer treatment a crime. Even though other American doctors were pleased to note her improved condition, "all they have to learn is that I went to Mexico for surgery and they look at me like a freak," she said.

It was within days of talking to Mrs. Clark that I met another outspoken Laetrile true believer, also in Concord: Mrs. Joan Wilkinson, a Denmark-born housewife and mother. In 1967, Mrs. Wilkinson said, she felt a growth in her left leg and also sensed "unusual heat" there. She had first been told there was nothing there, but she was later x-rayed and a growth was found on the bone. In her first U.S. operation, a tumor was removed from her leg. Two and a half months later she was back in the hospital with a malignancy necessitating the removal of muscle and bone.

Out of the hospital all was well for a time, but in 1968 she discovered a lump in the groin. Her doctor ordered a biopsy and she received the bad news: she had internal tumors of the lower abdomen. The doctors recommended amputation of her left leg and hip and other internal surgery. As Mrs. Wilkinson detailed it for *Prevention* magazine in December 1971:

> *The surgeon, who also happened to be the head of the Cancer Society, took a book off a shelf and very cruelly told me what parts of the body would have to be removed. He traced the leg and organs with a pencil on an illustration of the human body.*
>
> *He also told me that before amputating he would do an exploratory of the lungs, and if he found cancer there, he would not amputate. As my husband put it, they would sew me up and send me home to die.*
>
> *It was a pretty bad time for us. I couldn't sleep. I started praying. Something told me — as if it were God himself telling me — "this tragedy cannot happen to me." It was as if I were another person . . .*

The next morning, her sister, Mrs. Vera Murray of nearby Orinda, called her, literally pleading with her to see Dr. Ernst Krebs, Sr. in San Francisco. Then Mrs. Wilkinson remembered her sister had told her about Krebs and Laetrile the year before, but she had forgotten. With the prospect of massive amputation and surgery facing her, and with the prediction of a probable six-week survival anyway, she decided she had nothing to lose.

Dr. Krebs, Sr., still practicing though in his eighties, started giving Mrs. Wilkinson large Laetrile injections. The tumor first grew in size, then began to recede — after five weeks of injections she could no longer feel it, she said. She continued 10cc. injections three times a week, accompanied by a special diet, one avoiding all dairy products and anything made with white flour. "And I felt wonderful!" the attractive housewife said. "In fact, in August 1969 the doctor told me I needed no more injections. My x-rays were clear, showing that the tumor had shrunk, was apparently encased in scar tissue, and was not active."

When the surgeon under whose knife she had originally planned to go learned she would not be having surgery, he told her she had six to eight weeks to live — three months at the most — and even pleaded with her, she recalls. Since that time, five years before, Mrs. Wilkinson had been quite visibly healthy. When I interviewed her at her home, only some scar tissue in the left leg bore evidence of her brush-with-death ordeal. Her family doctor, she said, did not approve of her Laetrile treatment although he said, "I'm happy it worked for you.'"

By 1972, terminal cancer patients, learning about Laetrile by word of mouth and through the rapidly advancing Committee for Freedom of Choice in Cancer Therapy, were coming to California, visiting Dr. Richardson in his clinic, or travelling to Mexico where Dr. Contreras and an expanded staff were treating increasing numbers of cancer patients quite legally. Two of the Richardson cases I interviewed in 1973 are particularly noteworthy, for they demonstrated response, or seeming response, to massive Laetrile treatment and clearly opposed the best orthodox medical thinking of seasoned medical men. Even though, in both cases, death finally ensued, life had been prolonged, pain reduced, and temporary, dramatic improvement noted. In two of the three cases noted here, Dr. Richardson pointed out, death was due to complications rather than to the cancer itself. And in both of these the patients had been subjected to toxic traditional therapy before turning to Laetrile.

An Illinois woman, Mrs. Julius Butler, had been diagnosed as having cancer in 1970 and had undergone a complete hysterectomy. In August 1971 she began to notice back pains. She was informed that her cancer was back, and she began taking cobalt treatments, which continued through 1971, 1972, and part of 1973. Those close to her used terms like "cooked" and "dehydrated" to describe the fifty-nine-year-old Mrs. Butler's condition after intensive cobalt therapy.

In and out of the hospital with a deteriorating condition, she was finally given up by the doctors. "They said nothing more could be done for her, that an operation would kill her," Julius Butler recalled. By this time, she was down to seventy-five pounds and was suffering from adhesions and bowel obstructions. She was taking morphine every two hours. Her digestive system was almost entirely inoperative and she was clearly at death's door.

Julius Butler heard of Laetrile, and also knew Dr. Richardson. He told his doctors about it and they said that although it could not legally be procured in Illinois, they would "look into it" — a process which took ten days as the life of Opal Butler, racked by cancer and cobalt, continued to ebb. Then Mrs. Butler received a legal opinion from a hospital attorney: no dice. Laetrile could not be used in any way by that hospital, since reputation, let alone license, was at stake. "I was told to give up all hope," Mr. Butler told me. Doctors could only offer an experimental new legal drug, but aside from that actually suggested that "she be allowed to slip away," he said.

Mr. Butler contacted Dr. Richardson and made the arrangements for his extremely critical wife to be flown in a stretcher from Chicago to San Francisco. This was done in June 1973. Opposing the earlier advice against operating on her, Dr. Richardson ordered surgery for her bowel obstructions and adhesions, thus somewhat restoring the digestive tract. She was placed immediately on daily intravenous Laetrile injections. She spent two and a half weeks in the hospital. Released July 13, she was recuperating in a Berkeley motel when I first talked to her. "If you think I look like death warmed over now, you should have seen me when I got here to the Bay Area," she said with a smile and in a very weak voice.

Under the constant care of nurses, Mrs. Butler was eating more, regaining weight, and, most important, *no longer felt any pain*, and was off morphine. This condition persisted for months — dramatic evidence that somehow something was right with Laetrile. Abandoned by competent and qualified physicians as a terminal cancer patient, she was out of pain and seemingly recovering in Berkeley. Time had been bought, and I had to shake my head once again: was this just another coincidence? That Mrs. Butler ultimately died — not, as Dr. Richardson pointed out, of cancer, but of other complications — hardly detracted from the strong likelihood that she had received considerable benefit from the "worthless apricot-pit cancer cure."

In the same motel, which I came to call the "Laetrile Towers," was another dramatic Richardson patient — the combative seventy-year-old head of the New England Rally for God, Family and Country. Mrs. Anna McKinney, the mother of nine and wife of a physician, had been told in Boston in February 1973, she said, that "nothing could be done" for her bladder and intestinal cancer. "I was told I had less than a year to live," she recalled. In fact, she survived until summer 1974.

She visited Dr. Richardson in March and for eighteen days took 3cc. daily of Laetrile. After two months of treatment, she returned to New England, where a urologist who examined her was "amazed" at the regression of symptoms. "I felt better, but not well," she said. Even so, her family doctor was impressed at her general condition.

Back under Richardson's care in August, almost seven months following her gloomy diagnosis, she felt "one thousand percent better," she asserted. "My doctor still can't believe it. When I saw him back home, he asked me, 'Are you going to give credit to Laetrile, or to God?' I of course answered, 'To God.' "

The devoutly religious Mrs. McKinney had touched on a point that I had heard emphasized before — and which I would hear emphasized again and again — and which I can only consider a variable in certain cancer "control" cases: pure faith. Mrs. Butler, Mrs. Clark, and Mrs. McKinney, among my interviewees, and later Pam McDaniel and Betty Elder, all emphasized in their talks with me virtually unswerving religious faith.

There had been some other fairly spectacular examples of Laetrile use that I learned about in the Bay Area. A Pinole woman whose sister had died in 1964 after forty-three x-ray treatments had decided that if she ever had cancer s would go see Dr. Krebs, Sr. When she developed rectal cancer, she began receiving intramuscular injections of three grams three times a week, beginning in 1969. The pain left her and the lump diminished. She went without Laetrile for five weeks following the senior Krebs's retirement. The pain returned, excruciatingly, and she went to see Dr. Contreras in Tijuana. There she resumed Laetrile injections, taking nine grams a week for ten months. By June 1973 she said the limp her pain had caused had gone in six weeks, her strength had gradually returned and she went back to work as an Oakland seamstress. As of the summer of 1973 she was down to a single injection of three grams once a week.

A thirty-one-year-old San Rafael widow who underwent sixty cobalt treatments in two months and was hospitalized "ten or twelve" times for treatment of Hodgkins disease before hearing about Laetrile, visited Contreras in Tijuana in February 1972. Though the kindly medic held out no hope, she wanted treatment and got it — to the tune of 1,500 milligrams a day. She told *Let's Live* magazine in June 1973 that within a week her pain had subsided and she was "looking better."

At the same time, San Francisco insurance man Jay M. Hutchinson, founder of the Test Laetrile Now Committee, reported "control" of lymphosarcoma — fourth-stage terminal cancer — through Laetrile, enzymes, and a special diet. Hutchinson is himself a dramatic case. He recalled that his doctors called him a "walking malignancy." Initial tests had revealed cancer spread uniformly throughout his lymph system and bone marrow. Kaiser Hospital doctors said it would not respond to irradiation and recommended a combination of chemotherapy treatments, which they acknowledged could cause loss of hair, bone marrow depression, destruction of red blood corpuscles, and nausea.

Hutchinson's employer told him of a cousin who had become a Laetrile patient under Dr. Ernesto Contreras seven years before; the patient's face, disfigured after several surgeries for melanoma, had healed in three months. Very quickly Hutchinson was on the plane for Tijuana. For three weeks he received intravenous Laetrile injections in three-gram doses. Back in San Francisco, he began an oral dosage of one and a half grams per day. This he continued for two months. After the third month he took a gram of Laetrile a day.

As he told *Let's Live* and confirmed to me personally:

Laetrile is the only thing I've taken, and I've had a year completely free from ailment.

I can't say Laetrile has produced the stabilized condition. All I can say is I am stabilized — it may be the diet, or a combination of both. There have been no further symptoms.

I have seen Dr. Contreras five times, and continue seeing my Kaiser physicians. Their medical reports contain the data on my Laetrile intake. The swelling is still there, but no larger. Sometimes it goes down to half-size for a while. There is no pain or discomfort.

In 1974 he had had almost three years free of disease

By 1973 the dam was bursting on "known" Laetrile and amygdalin therapy cases in the United States. Dr. John A. Richardson said he had treated 750 patients with Laetrile as part of his basic megavitamin therapy. In all cases palliation, ranging from minimal and temporary to considerable and longterm, had occurred.

By 1976, the Richardson clinic had treated up to 6,000 persons with total megavitamin therapy for cancer, with Dr. Richardson reporting a better than 60-percent "positive response" ratio, certainly in keeping with the statistics of Dr. Ernesto Contreras in Mexico, Dr. Paul Wedel of Oregon, and a growing number of Laetrile-using practitioners around the country.

Dr. Wedel, a metabolic therapist who ranks among the best in the world, became known to the Committee for Freedom of Choice in 1975, and by 1976 had treated some 4,000 people with Laetrile and related therapies. Dr. Wedel's situation is unusually significant since he himself is a Laetrile recovery patient.

Dr. Lawrence McDonald of Atlanta, Georgia, who had been a skeptic but who became more convinced about Laetrile efficacy after attending a Laetrile seminar in January 1973, went on to become a Laetrile and freedom-of-choice-defending U.S. Congressman. Both as a urologist and a federal congressman he testified in behalf of Dr. Richardson during the latter's trials. He was also on hand as an "expert witness" in other Laetrile-connected litigation. At the time of the Richardson trials Dr. McDonald testified he had treated 80 patients in Atlanta with Laetrile therapy — and with no legal consequences, since Georgia has no specific statutes barring use of the substance. The McDonald success ratio was about the same as Richardson's.

At the Richardson trials I met several dozen more cancer "controllees" — members and supporters of the Committee for Freedom of Choice in Cancer Therapy, all of them prior or ongoing patients of Dr. Hans Nieper in West Germany, Dr. Ernesto Contreras in Tijuana, or Dr. Richardson in California.

A Millbrae, California, grandmother reported on a controlled leukemia case, that of her four-year-old grandson, in a letter to Sloan-Kettering's Dr. Kanematsu Sugiura, who was conducting the Laetrile tests at the prestigious institute from 1973 to 1975. On December 13, 1973. Mrs. Lynn Conragan wrote in part:

> *Kindly note copy of the enclosed letter (hospital analysis of her grandson done July 15, 1970). The child in question is my grandson who will be four years old in three weeks and is the picture of health. Yet we were told, when he was three months of age, that he would live only at the most an additional 30 days!*
>
> *Shaun, my grandson, was born with leukemia — yet the physicians treated my daughter like another hysterical new mother when she tried to tell them the first three months of his life that the child was ill and not responding normally to food, etc....*
>
> *We physically took this child out of the hospital over the attending physicians' protest and, knowing we had nothing to lose, started him immediately on Laetrile and 500 mg. daily of every high-powered vitamin that we could get into him, such as C, E, Wheat Germ, enzymes, etc....*
>
> *My grandson has had no chemotherapy since he was 10 months of age and no irradiation therapy to the spleen since 3 months of age....*
>
> *My only despair is the thought of all the infants I saw in the hospital with the same disease, at the same time as Shaun, who were*

*experimented upon by well-meaning physicians, but are now dead
because the medical profession itself is still in a self-imposed darkness.*[1]

And Marcia Laurence, of San Carlos, California, wrote Sloan-
Kettering's Dr. Lloyd Old on July 15, 1973, concerning her amazing case
treated by Dr. Nieper:

> *I am writing at the behest of Dr. Hans Nieper of Hannover, Ger-
> many, to whom I went for cancer therapy in February of this year. I am
> overjoyed that someone of your stature in American cancer investigation
> might be interested in my case history, because it is my firm belief that
> Dr. Nieper's therapy saved my life. I believe, likewise, that countless other
> lives could be saved if the same therapy were recognized and practiced in
> the United States . . .*
>
> *Approximately 8 years ago I discovered a lump in my right breast
> which was diagnosed as carcinoma and which was excised by a radical
> mastectomy. Three months later I submitted to a single mastectomy of
> the left breast upon the recommendation of the cancer board of the
> hospital which was based on the history of breast cancer on both sides of
> my family, my young age (35), the significant incidence of transference of
> tumor from one breast to the other, and the fact that my tumor, unlike
> the majority, appeared in the right breast. I had had my uterus removed
> after my last C Section, but no oophorectomy was recommended. I
> recovered and had no trouble of this nature for seven years.*
>
> *In May of 1972 I had an anterior spinal fusion at C-5, C-6.
> Following this, my neck pain at first subsided and then began to build in
> intensity until I had to be readmitted to the hospital. X-rays revealed
> lesions involving vertebrae C-2 through C-5. I was sent to Stanford to
> begin radiation on the Linear Accelerator and to have an oophorectomy.*
>
> *I had maximum radiation to my entire spine, and, because my neck
> was in such bad shape, I needed to roll in bed from my back to my side for
> several weeks. Shortly after starting radiation, an oophorectomy was per-
> formed.*
>
> *At the end of July I was discharged to continue my recuperation at
> home and continue radiation as an out-patient. Although I was free of
> neck pain, I could not hold my head up for very long as my neck was too
> weak to support it. Also, I was so debilitated that the most simple actions
> became major efforts most of which I did not have the stamina to per-
> form. I need to interject here that when the oophorectomy was performed,
> it was found that the peritoneum was studded with tumor. There were
> nodules on the right ovary and over the liver.*
>
> *In January, 1973, pain erupted in my right upper arm and x-rays
> revealed tumor in the humerus. I was sent immediately into radiation*

(4,000 rads). The surgical department then began talking seriously about an adrenalectomy, while the radiation department recommended chemotherapy, the time to start being discretionary with the surgical department.

It was at this point that my husband and I drew a halt to the proceedings. From Dr. Victor Richards' book The Wayward Cell *we had learned that the prognoses for the American cancer therapies for metastases (were) very far from encouraging. We also read a quote of Dr. Frank Rauscher Jr. that only about 7 ½ percent of all human cancers of (metastatic) nature can be brought to the status of 5-year survival. When I asked one of my doctors at Stanford for my prognosis, he simply told me to live one day at a time. My body had deteriorated to such an extent that I arranged to leave my body to the University and my eyes to the Eye Bank. I still wore my cervical collar 75 percent of the time, spinal pressure somewhere kept my right hand perpetually tingly and numb, and I wore my right arm in a sling, although I had been warned that because the humerus was so thin my arm would, in all likelihood, fracture spontaneously.*

We had heard Dr. Dean Burk speak of Laetrile over television. We heard more in-depth discussion of it at a symposium of the International Assn. of Cancer Victims and Friends which we attended as members.

After questioning several members and doctors there, including Dr. Burk, we decided to see Dr. Nieper in Germany. At this time we had little real faith that the progress of my metastases might be stopped; we simply felt that we must look outside the United States for assistance in bringing me to a state of some health so that whatever survival time I had remaining might be spent in as near normal a way as was possible.

In the United States cancer therapy consists of cutting, burning or poisoning. I did not feel I could afford to be decimated further as already each day for me was something of an ordeal.

In February, I flew over to see Dr. Nieper. When I left, I was wearing my collar, my sling, and I had to be transported to the plane in a wheel chair as I was too weak to walk the distance required. I saw the doctor on weekdays for slightly less than three weeks, and my husband and I took another four weeks coming home at a leisurely pace.

By the time I arrived home, I was not only strongly walking long distances without tiring. I was carrying my own luggage without difficulty, and I felt in better health than I had felt in at least ten years!

While I was with the doctor, extremely severe pain in my right side indicated the presence of metastasis (which, had I been in this country, would have sent me into radiation forthwith). Dr. Nieper told me it was something I should disregard for the present; the pain was severe for about a week, it was at a fairly tolerable level for another week, by the third week the pain was only spasmodic, and thereafter I forgot I'd had it.

X-rays taken upon my return to Stanford revealed metastases in right ribs 10 and 11 but the condition appeared to be stabilized and the absence of pain dictated against radiation therapy. Another test indicated the absence of metastasis in my liver. My examination at Stanford revealed me to be in good shape with relation to the cancer, and it was noted that my "general feeling of well being is outstanding."[2]

Mrs. Laurence described the Nieper treatment, which the West German medic relayed via a tape recording for her stateside doctors. The specific cancer-cell destroyer prescribed was amygdalin. He also prescribed numerous other medications for metabolic therapy, bone recalcification, and other processes, as well as a strict diet.

Like so many others, the Laurence case was a losing battle against cancer, but to Mrs. Laurence the positive aspect of the treatment was the noticeable reduction in pain and suffering and the restoration of a sense of well-being. Too, she was obviously surviving longer than American orthodox medicine would have predicted.

Again and again I was learning of palliation from amygdalin therapy. If such therapy provided nothing more than relief from pain, why, *why* did it remain illegal for use in cancer therapy?

In California Superior Court testimony of 1976, Dr. James Privitera, who had been arrested twice in 1975 with vitamin distributors on a variety of Laetrile-connected charges, and a group of whose patients tried unsuccessfuly to enjoin the state from banning his use of vitamin B-17 in their cases, testified about twenty-two Laetrile-vitamin therapy cases this way:

Every one of the 22 patients or survivors of patients testified to the dramatic improvement in sense of well-being, increased appetite, gain in weight and reduction in pain. These four improvements have been significantly noted by me in practically every patient having cancer that I have seen in my office since beginning the use of the dietary program which I have developed and advocate for such patients.

In this dietary program the amygdalin (vitamin B-17) is the keystone for the patient having cancer because we almost invariably see, associated with it, an improvement in the sense of well-being, increase in appetite, gain in weight and decrease in pain. In the absence of amygdalin the patient having cancer does not dramatically improve in the sense of well-being, increased appetite or weight gain, and there is seldom any decrease in the amount of pain present, irrespective of the fact that all other nutritional ingredients in the program are administered.

Although no score sheet on a patient-by-patient basis has been kept I can state conservatively that at least 70 percent of all my patients who have cancer have experienced very substantial or dramatic improvements in all of the four categories of improvement just mentioned, and up to 90 percent of all such patients improve to some extent at least, or even substantially, in one or more of such categories of improvement.[3]

When interviewing the Laetrile patients, hearing about Laetrile cases, perusing the earlier information on Laetrile and amygdalin, it seemed to me a pattern was forming, one not susceptible of an offhand putdown by governmental decree. Laetrile obviously was having a positive effect in a huge number of cases. Often, it was clearly associated with spectacular effects. No one in the front rank of the Laetrile movement — not Ernst Krebs, Jr., not Dr. Contreras, not Andrew McNaughton, not Dean Burk — was talking about the infallibility of Laetrile. There were dead Laetrile patients as well as live ones. No one talked cure; the most I ever heard in terms of claims was the word "control." No doctor involved in the Laetrile story was claiming vitamin B-17 was the last, final word. And even Krebs, while wholeheartedly dedicated to the unitarian trophoblastic theory of cancer, continually stressed that the substance did one thing and one thing only in cancer therapy; it inhibited cancer tumors. It could not restore destroyed tissues.

The fact that patients might take Laetrile and still die of cancer was used repeatedly to discredit Laetrile — yet never used to discredit 5-Fu, methotrexate, or any "orthodox" poison. For the great majority of American cancer patients have been treated with such "orthodox" methods — and eventually died.

Two California cancer cases in which the patients were reportedly treated only with Laetrile alone and then died were brought up at a cancer congress in Toronto, Canada, in May 1976, though no details of either case were revealed in the press.

At the same congress, the seemingly incessant controversy over the Sloan-Kettering mouse tests continued as one of the researchers who had failed to replicate Dr. Sugiura's experiments testified that "all evidence shows conclusively that Laetrile is without anti-cancer properties."

This utter misstatement was similar to such global utterances as "without a shred of evidence" and "utterly worthless" as adduced by the American Cancer Society and Food and Drug Administration in the 1970s to dismiss Laetrile. The foregoing case histories put the lie to such global assessments as to the worthlessness of vitamin B-17.

But by 1976, and despite the mixed results on mouse cancer, there were the beginnings of evidence that vitamin B-17 therapy could be useful in domesticated cats and dogs as well. Improvements were noted in both varieties of animals — improvements which could hardly be attributed to "subjective response" or the "placebo effect."

California veterinarian John E. Craige reported, in *Feline Practice* for June 1976, on the positive effects from the use of vitamin B-17 in the treatment of cats suffering from leukemia and leukemia-like symptoms. In the June and July issues of *The Choice*, Dr. Craige reported he had found positive effects in three cats suffering from leukemia, had seen positive effects on ten other cats exhibiting leukemia-like symptoms, and then revealed in detail the incredible, if temporary, metabolic response of a prize-winning Norwegian elkhound to Laetrile therapy.

In 1974, veterinarian George Browne, Jr. reported on total remission of a thyroid cancer in a male Pekinese dog.[4]

In all of these cases, Laetrile was used as an injectable, or in tablet form, or as natural vitamin B-17 in apricot kernels.

Just as in the cases of the humans involved, the animals showed responses to vitamin B-17, including restoration of appetite, gain in weight, and/or demonstrable increase in friskiness.

Dr. Craige reported in 1976 that a virtual epidemic of leukemia was sweeping through the domesticated cat population in the United States. Why would domesticated dogs and cats be showing up with a cancer epidemic? In accordance with the vitamin-deficiency and dietary theory of cancer, one would reach the same conclusion as the Laetrilists speculate for humans.

The diet of domesticated dogs and cats is as processed, tampered with, denaturalized and stripped of a number of useful vitamins and ingredients as is the diet of "civilized" man.

How else explain the frequent tableau of cancer-stricken dogs, cats and humans on an American farm, living and working in the presence of non-cancer-stricken *grazing* animals? Following the viral theory of cancer, such a setting presents us with the unlikely reality of a *domestic*, or "house-oriented" virus. Carcinogenic contaminants in the atmosphere must be discarded since all farm animals are exposed to the same environment. So either a domestic virus is involved — or, more rationally and most obviously, the difference is in what the humans, the domesticated dogs and cats, and the grazing farm animals are *eating*.

The farm animals are apt to be on an entirely natural whole diet of grazing grasses (Johnson or sudan, for example) and in so doing receive enormous portions of vitamin B-17. The humans and their domesticated dogs and cats are surviving on "enriched," unnatural, processed, tampered-with manufactured foods almost totally lacking in the vitamin.

There is nothing in the above cases of both humans and domesticated animals to suggest that vitamin B-17 (Laetrile) is the single, one-and-only answer in the *treatment* of cancer, but there is growing evidence that it is the preventative substance *par excellence* in heading off the disease.

As we will explore in further chapters, there is controversy among laetrilists themselves as to how Laetrile "works" — and there are obvious cases in which it is "working" little if at all in *treating* cancer. Yet a total metabolic treatment program stressing vitamins, enzymes and diet in which vitamin B-17 plays the central role does appear, at this time, as the most biologically reasonable approach to cancer — particularly if it is borne in mind that Laetrile therapy may be used with "orthodox" therapy.

The most exciting aspect of the Laetrile story is not, however, in the treatment of cancer. It is in the possibility of the elimination of this scourge in a single generation, through a dietary revolution and the return, in our eating habits, of adequate levels of vitamin B-17.

CHAPTER FOUR

The Battle of Unorthodoxy

THERE IS NOTHING NEW about challenges to scientific orthodoxy, challenges which shake the very foundations of conventional wisdom. Indeed, the history of scientific breakthroughs is one of repeated unorthodox challenges to orthodox articles of faith. Laetrile, or vitamin B-17, is only one in a series of such challenges. And without a doubt it is the most serious challenge to orthodox thinking about cancer.

The frontiers of science are usually explored by persons with unorthodox approaches. Copernicus and Galileo had the brassbound gall to assert that a ro id world went around the sun. They flew in the face of conventional wisdom and mightily ruffled the feathers of the theological-scientific establishment of their day. Sir Alexander Fleming once noted that penicillin stayed on the shelf for years while orthodox medicine condemned him as a quack, a deceiver of the public. Lister, Harvey, Semmelweiss, and Pasteur were all, in their time, thought to be quacks or ignored as they forged new frontiers in science and medicine.

Medical orthodoxy has played key roles in history; for centuries, for example, "bleeding" was the standard treatment for a host of conditions. George Washington was bled four times in a twelve-hour period for treatment of a cold. The very weakened father of his country was then administered calomel and huge doses of tartar emetic. Moreover, pulverized beetles were put around his neck to raise blisters. Everything failed and he died of pneumonia.

Perhaps the most widely reported death of a monarch — and the most vivid description of orthodox medical practice in the seventeenth century — was the passing of King Charles II of England; eight detailed versions of his demise are extant and come from the pens of doctors and other witnesses. That the well-meaning attending physicians helped speed the death of the monarch is, with the security of hindsight, beyond a reasonable doubt. What they did to poor Charles!

Sir Charles Scarburgh, Charles II's personal physician, informs us that on February 2, 1685, the monarch suddenly suffered a loss of speech and went into convulsions.[1] Immediately two physicians drew out sixteen ounces of blood from his right arm, applied cupping glasses to his shoulders and "scarification deep enough to effect a fuller and more vigorous revulsion," thereby drawing off an additional eight ounces of blood. To free his stomach and digestive system from "impurities," the physicians next administered an emetic consisting of "orange infusion of the metals, made in white wine," white vitriol, and peony water. This was followed by an enema made of powder of sacred bitters, syrup of buckthorn, rock salt, and more of the orange infusion of metals. "Above and byond this, so as to leave no stone unturned, blistering agents were applied all over his head, after his hair had been shaved."

Special preparations followed "to give strength to his loaded brain" (sacred bitters powder, peony water, bryony compound) and to "excite sneezing," with powder of white hellebore roots "to be applied to the King's nostrils as occasion arose." A second brain strengthener (four ounces of cowslip flowers) was added, as were a preparation (manna, barley water, cream of tartar) to "keep his bowels active at night" and an emulsion of barley, licorice, and sweet almond kernels to "counteract the scalding of his urine, likely to result from the use of blistering drugs."

While he was fed these remedies and broths, "spirit of sal ammoniac was applied now and again to His Most Serene Majesty's nostrils" along with another substance, and "cephalic plasters combined with spurge and burgundy pitch, in equal parts, were applied to the soles of his feet."

These same general procedures continued on February 3, with an additional ten ounces of blood removed from his jugular vein and a new emulsion administered to counteract scalding of the urine. The king now complained of a sore throat and for this a special mixture for gargling was provided, consisting of inner bark of elm, barley water, and syrup of mallow. A julep of various sweeteners was then prescribed.

On February 4 a "mild laxative" consisting of white tartar, white wine, senna leaves, manna, flowers of chamomile, gentian root, and nutmeg was administered. These remedies failed to do the trick, and Scarburgh notes that "as His Serene Majesty's condition became most grave as the night advanced, the physicians who were watching him considered it advisable to administer the following small draught — B. spirit of human skull, 40 drops."

On February 5, to counteract a fever, the body of physicians provided Peruvian bark, antidotal milk water, and syrup of cloves. They continued using extract of human skull in a "pearl julep." Yet on February 6, "as the illness was now becoming more grave and His Most Serene Majesty's strength (Woe's me!) gradually failing, the physicians were compelled to have recourse to the more active cardiac tonics, and to prescribe the following . . . Raleigh's stronger antidote," an essence of dissolved pearl, and goa stone. A host of remedies followed during the day, including more sal ammoniac and bezoar stones from animal intestines. All of these measures failed to alleviate the Royal Personage's condition, and at length Charles II expired.

Raymond Crawfurd, having researched the illness and treatment of Charles II, concludes that actually the malady was a form of Bright's disease and that the misuse of the blistering agents — Spanish fly, or cantharides — proved fatal, robbing the kidneys of their last vestige of functional activity. The point here is that the best medical thinking of the century was marshaled in defense of Charles II's last hours. That thinking probably killed him.

In the matter of cancer in the twentieth century, orthodox medicine is faced with a severe challenge: the disease, in any of its officially cited 100 basic forms (or its varying 200 — or even more — forms), has reached epidemic proportions in the Western world and in most technological and industrialized countries elsewhere. By 1976 the death rate from cancer was accelerating at the fastest pace in 25 years of statistics-keeping, according to the American Cancer Society and the National Cancer Institute.

The orthodox approach to cancer remains surgery, x-rays, radioactive substances, and various toxic chemotherapeutic compounds and hormones, with a small but growing interest in immunotherapy — that is, stimulating the body's own immunosuppressive system to help combat cancer. All of these approaches are based on treatment rather than prevention and, with the possible exception of the as-yet infant interest in immunotherapy, constitute methods that are so marginally effective that no optimistic assault on cancer incidence and death-rate statistics has been made, as we will show.

At some point, governmental power and medical practice began to fuse in this country, so much so, indeed, that by "medical establishment" one tended to mean the points of view of the powerful American Medical Association and the enforcing, enabling capacities of the Food and Drug Administration. Persons who tended to run afoul of the scientific bases and conventional wisdom of the AMA usually found themselves in hot water with state departments of public health and the FDA.

In fact, unorthodox researchers and scientists, and in general nutritional experts who believe much of established medicine in America is based on unnatural (that is, drug) approaches to prevention and treatment rather than on natural ones (food, nutrition, etc.), have denounced the medical establishment with such terms as "medical politicians" and have spoken of a medical-governmental-pharmaceutical monopoly intent on peddling pills and expensive drugs to an American public that is getting progressively sicker.

In the area of cancer, researchers who deviated from conventional wisdom — and little wisdom about the complex of diseases called cancer can actually be described as conventional — were vigorously harassed by the medical profession and established law. We are not here jumping to conclusions as to the efficacy or lack thereof of the unorthodox or "unproven" methods of cancer treatment, but we refer to them in passing — for each and every one of them ran up against a solid wall of opposition and generally involved assaults on their proponents' character, lengthy litigation, and, for all intents and purposes, defeat.

Dr. Max Gerson, a highly respected M.D., was one of the first of the metabolic therapy pioneers to note the connection between nutrition and cancer. In the 1940s and 1950s he advanced case after case to indicate that a radical change in nutrition, accompanied by a vigorous detoxification program, constituted the probable answer to the treatment of cancer. But he was maligned for such "heresy," damned as a nutritional quack, and even declared a fraud by the New York County Medical Society. Those who did not read beyond the headlines were unaware that Albert Schweitzer, who credited Dr. Gerson with saving his wife's life, called him a "medical genius who walked among us." Dr. Gerson's daughter has continued to advance his work.

Dr. William S. Koch, who advanced a substance called Glyoxylide in cancer therapy, fought medical orthodoxy and governmental bureaucracy for more than two decades in the United States, all the while being damned as a quack, while some 2,000 osteopaths and naturopaths pointed to benefits from use of the substance. Dr. Koch eventually left — or, as some insist, was "driven from" — the country to continue his work. There are cancer recovery patients today who still claim they owe their lives to the "Koch agents" — Glyoxylide and related substances, some of which are still used in metabolic therapy.

Overlapping the Koch and Gerson era (pre-World War II and the first decades thereafter) was the national furor over Krebiozen, a substance originally advanced by Yugoslav scientists but particularly championed in this country by one of America's most respected orthodox physicians, Dr. Andrew C. Ivy of the University of Illinois. Though this simple, inexpensive, apparently non-toxic cancer treatment at one time had nearly 20,000 testimonial case histories in its defense, and although Dr. Ivy was one of the best-credentialed cancer researchers in the country, the government and the medical establishment went to extraordinary lengths to destroy both Krebiozen — later sold in this country as Carcalon — and Dr. Ivy. The federal government unleashed a multi-million-dollar prosecution against Ivy, his colleagues and Krebiozen, which lasted 289 days, included testimony which the government later admitted was falsified, and a vigorous campaign by the anti-Krebiozen lobby in the press. Neither the FDA nor the American Cancer Society like to recall that, despite all of the hoopla over this allegedly quack cancer cure, this "unproven remedy," the four defendants were all eventually acquitted of the 240 counts against them. And, the jury even added that it believed the substance involved had merit — a proper conclusion to reach following a string of well-documented testimony as to its efficacy. Yet the propaganda campaign paid off, and Krebiozen was left in the public mind as another unproven cancer remedy and Dr. Ivy was character-assassinated into the limbo reserved for pioneers who dare operate outside of the medical-governmental axis.

What had happened?

Benedict F. Fitzgerald, Jr., special counsel to the Committee on Interstate and Foreign Commerce, came the closest to revealing in public what actually lay behind the persecution not only of Krebiozen, but also of the almost equally popular "unproven remedy," the Hoxsey herbal preparations. In a report to the Senate Interstate Commerce Committee on the Need for the Investigation of Cancer Research Organizations and carried in the *Congressional Record* of August 28, 1953, pp. 5690-93, we find in Fitzgerald's report:

> *I have concluded that in the value of present cancer research, this substance (Krebiozen) and the theory behind it deserve the most full and complete and scientific study. Its value in the management of the cancer patient has been demonstrated in a sufficient number and percentage of cases to demand further work. Behind and over all this is the weirdest conglomeration of corrupt motives, intrigue, selfishness, jealousy, obstruction, and conspiracy that I have ever seen.*

Fitzgerald found the same to be true in the matter of the Hoxsey approach, and in his report we read that "the jury, after listening to leading pathologists, radiologists, physicians, surgeons, and scores of witnesses, a great number of whom had never been treated by any physician or surgeon except the treatment received at the Hoxsey Cancer Clinic, concluded that Dr. (Morris) Fishbein (of the American Medical Assn.) was wrong; that his published statements were false, and that the Hoxsey method of treating cancer did have therapeutic value."

Moreover, the report continued:

> *. . . We should determine whether existing agencies, both public and private, are engaged and have pursued a policy of harassment, ridicule, slander, and libelous attacks on others sincerely engaged in stamping out*

this curse of mankind. Have medical associations, through their officers, agents, servants and employees, engaged in this practice? My investigation to date should convince this committee that a conspiracy does exist to stop the free flow and use of drugs in interstate commerce which allegedly (have) therapeutic value. Public and private funds have been thrown around like confetti at a country fair to close up and destroy clinics, hospitals, and scientific research laboratories which do not conform to the viewpoint of medical associations.

Additionally, Fitzgerald pointed to the cancer-causing potential of X-ray treatment in cancer, being promoted then (as now, along with chemotherapy) as the best approach in cancer therapy.

Hence, though Dr. Ivy's Krebiozen and Harry Hoxsey's herbal treatments actually won their days in court after enormous expenditures for the defendants, enough damage was brought by a powerful convergence of forces to convince the public that both were nothing more than quackery. Accordingly, Krebiozen was almost blitzed out of existence, and the Hoxsey treatment fell from its gathering popularity (although as of this writing it is still available in Tijuana, Mexico). There remain today thousands of adherents who claim positive results from both approaches.

For his efforts, FitzGerald was reportedly "summarily discharged" after filing his report — the first "official" recognition of an organized conspiracy to stamp out unwanted cancer remedies.

Laetrile — that is, its modern form — was developed at the time of the Hoxsey and Krebiozen furors. Suppressed early in its life, the substance did not come into its own until a quarter-century later, and then almost entirely because it became the center of a major political, let alone scientific, controversy. It was on the way to being suppressed out of existence, intermittently kept alive by The McNaughton Foundation and by a small band of harassed clinicians and scientists around the world, until the advent of the Richardson arrest and the full-scale entry into the controversy by John Birch Society members, who perceived in the Laetrile matter the overriding issue of the trampling on freedom of choice by governmental force. Hence Laetrile was to become the single "unorthodox, unproven cancer remedy" in this country which went on the offensive and began winning acceptance in an unparalleled struggle involving grass roots organizing, politicking and counter-propaganda. It also remained, of all the "unorthodox" remedies, the one most widely and scientifically supported.

It is neither the scope nor intent of this book to make a case for any of the above-described "unproven cancer remedies," or even to go into much detail as to presumptive conspiracy theories as they relate to cancer. The Birch Society members battling within the movement have already done yeoman work in the latter area, particularly G. Edward Griffin in *World Without Cancer*. In the work, which is available both as a filmstrip and as a book, Griffin points to an economic wedding between Rockefeller and German interests which constructed a vast drug and pharmaceutical cartel, one which paralleled a tenuous if powerful collaborative effort at world government and an overlap with monopolies in a variety of industries.

What is the situation today?

As of the 1970s, conditions globally referred to as "degenerative diseases" — the complex of illnesses jointly called "heart disease" ranking first; cancer, in second place (although cancer is now the number-one killer of children in the United States); the "silent" precursor conditions, including hypertension, arteriosclerosis, and hypoglycemia; diabetes, perhaps cystic fibrosis and a variety of lesser maladies — constitute far and away the great majority of admissions to hospitals and clinics. Their victims are the most frequent customers of the "health-care delivery industry." That is to say, diseases produced by bacteria and parasites are no longer the major threat to the nation's health. It can be said that traditional Western medicine has done an excellent job in stamping out or greatly limiting the great infectious killers of mankind, to the extent that such infectious killers other than venereal disease (whose pandemicity is due not to scientific ineptitude but to the breakdown in morals which characterizes much of the "civilized" world) are virtually forgotten and hardly to be feared.

However, medical orthodoxy approaches the degenerative diseases as if they were infectious states — hence the multibillion-dollar hunt for the "human, cancer-causing virus." And orthodoxy treats the diseases as if they were infections — hence the development of expensive, toxic drugs and the reliance on "cut, burn and poison" (radical surgery, radiation and-or chemotherapy in cancer, and surgery and potent drugs in heart disease). The fact that the Western World now has a major epidemic of both cancer and heart disease constitutes the best evidence that our scientific premises about the degenerative diseases are basically in error, and that cut-burn-and-poison not only is not making a statistical dent in the incidence of these diseases, but very likely is helping spread them.

Interlocked with this reality is the continual reliance upon surgery as medicine's *creme de la creme*, when it is now estimated that billions of dollars are spent needlessly in this country on surgery that either was unnecessary or, even worse, has a negative effect on the patient.

Another significant result is the accruing of vast profits to the drug industry, an industry based on, or simply conveniently intertwined with, the current false medical premises regarding the degenerative diseases. As reported in 1976 in *Town and Country's* thorough research into nutrition, vitamins and the modern diseases, such a common substance as Valium, which was dispensed 22.5 million times in this country in 1974, at an average of 60 tablets per prescription — for a total of 1 billion, 350 million tablets sold — was being sold at an enormous profit. The cost per kilo in Switzerland is estimated at $50, while the cost per kilo in this country soars to $75,000 before the tablets are ready for sale. Assuming similar multi-thousand-percent markups for the full range of drugs, compounds, and substances used in heart disease and cancer, which together account for some 70 percent of fatalities per year in the United States, we are looking at a gargantuan drug and medicine industry *based on the reality, if not the hope, of people getting sicker, not healthier.*

Also interlocked in this picture is yet another reality: the conglomerate of interests called the "food-processing industry," certainly beginning with but not limited to processed white sugar and processed white flour. It is perhaps *the* major industry in the United States today, and the disastrous American diet of processed, denaturalized, conserved, preserved, chemically treated and often polluted foods is being ever more suspiciously viewed as the *primary* cause of degenerative diseases (rather than bacteria, viruses and infectious states). In the entire food-processing picture we are looking at multiples of billions of dollars in investments and certainly millions of jobs.

Now, along come the naturopaths, homeopaths, assorted vitamin and diet fanatics and the growing if tiny field of metabolic or "holistic" medical therapists who believe that the degenerative diseases are not caused *by* something but by a *lack* of something. The lack, they say, is proper diet and man's wholesale departure from biological and evolutionary common sense through ingestion of a "civilized" diet almost totally at variance with man's original "natural" diet. These practitioners are in effect saying that the medicine of the future is prevention, not treatment, and that the killer diseases of civilization are amenable to prevention through proper diet and a return to biological sanity in the foods we eat; and that, in terms of treatment, dietary manipulation and therapy based on vitamins, minerals and enzymes are *the answer.*

Preventive medicine is a threat of enormous dimensions to therapeutic medicine. It means the ultimate removal of the vast amount of degenerative disease cases from the rolls of hospitals and clinics, the great majority of whose admissions are degenerative disease cases. In the meantime, vitamins, minerals and "health foods" pose a threat of equal magnitude to the food-processing industry and to the international drug cartel. The federal government's conclusion that the profits of the health food and vitamin industry in this country as of 1975 ran in excess of $400 million is a statistic which pales alongside the incalculable billions of dollars of investment in, and profit from, the threatened food processing industry and the pharmaceutical monopolies whose simple substances are marked up by the *thousands* of percent over actual costs of raw materials.

As of 1972, *California Business* reported (Nov. 9, 1972) that cancer as a "business," based on median costs per patient, was a $12-billion-per-year expenditure (or profit). These figures have been estimated upward since that time in amounts ranging from $16 to $20 billion per year (items: hospital rooms per day, internal medicine, anesthesia, drugs, surgery, medical insurance, doctor visits, all associated with cancer), and by 1975 officialdom set the price tag on cancer (including the cost to the country through man-hours lost to industry through cancer) at around $25 billion. It is fair to say that cancer now constitutes an industry in excess of $20 billion. But cancer is only the *tip* of the degenerative disease iceberg: throw in heart disease in all its forms, and allied degenerative disease conditions, and we are dealing with expenditures and profits which surely range well beyond $100 billion.[2]

If it can be demonstrated, as the vitamin B-17 proponents are demonstrating, that cancer is, basically, a vitamin-deficiency disease, amenable to metabolic and nutritional treatment (aside from being *preventable* through maintenance of an adequate diet and sufficient levels of vitamin B-17 in the system), then the cancer industry itself is in peril. If the cancer industry is imperiled, the entire card house of the degenerative disease industry collapses. There would be a domino effect which ultimately would pose a gigantic threat to the pharmaceutical monopolies, the international drug cartel and even the food-processing industry.

All of this must be seen as a powerful, if not overriding, reason behind the suppression of unwanted, uncontrolled or outside-the-pale medical remedies. Herein may very well lie part of the "conspiracy" which Birchers have long warned about.

How vested interests, ego concerns, and simple economics and politics might merge to muddy the already befouled waters about cancer — its control, cure, and prevention — is an ever-recurring question that admits of no single answer. And the Birchers, arriving late in the Laetrile story, were by no means the first to raise it.

Morris A. Bealle, who wrote on medical and pharmaceutical matters, was perhaps one of the most informed and outspoken observers of what he called the "drug trust," an interlocking web of pharmaceutical houses which in turn is said to overlap with established medicine and governmental agencies. He detailed "the largest drug manufacturing combine in the world," which he attributed to Eastern interests, and charged that the combine uses all its other interests "to bring pressure to continue and increase the sale of drugs."[3]

In *Super Drug Story* he also insisted that "not only does the F.D.A. wink at violations by the Drug Trust . . . but it is very assiduous in putting out of business any and all vendors of therapeutic devices which increase the healthy incidence of the public and thus decrease the profit incidence of the Drug Trust." The bureau "is used primarily for the perversion of justice by 'cracking down' on all who endanger the profits of the Drug Trust," he adds, claiming that the alleged trust sees vitamins as a key threat to profits, and argues that the American Medical Association is little more than a "powerful subsidiary of the Drug Trust." He then quotes Dr. Emanuel M. Josephson:

> *Associations have been formed to "control cancer." They have been more successful in controlling the cancer business. If they incidentally increase the financial returns on their doctors' investments in radium — it must be said that the price of radium increased 1,000 percent when they began to use it on cancer victims — that was hardly unexpected or undesired.*
>
> *These doctors proclaim themselves "authorities" and "specialists" in cancer. They systematically deny everything that does not emanate from themselves and add to their cash incomes. Since these fakers would be "robbed" of their livelihoods and incomes by any effective means of preventing cancer, they can be depended on to promptly reject any method which might be discovered. As "omniscient authorities" they vehemently scorn and discredit any such possibility. They happily insist that the cancer problem will be with us forever.*
>
> *Cancer associations do not use the funds they collect for the relief of cancer victims or for the payment of institutions for their care. The money collected has been used for the payment of salaries to the medical bosses, to other personnel and for publicity, propaganda and advertising (for more contributions).*

In the meantime, Americans have been fed the collectivistic line that their government somehow protects them from fraud, bad drugs and bad food. If only it were so!

The Food and Drug Administration (FDA), as the policing arm of the food and drug industries, may from time to time have cracked down on authentically worthless nostrums and certain interstate frauds, but the fact it also doubles as a "Fedstapo" for the medical-pharmaceutical-monopoly axis can hardly be denied. If the FDA bureaucracy, swollen in size and duties, constitutes "the watchers," then, as the saying goes, "who will watch the watchers?"

It is through FDA rules and regulations — with or without any real force in law — that Laetrile and/or any other unwanted or threatening remedy is "kept off the market." By sheer dint of bureaucracy (see Chapter 7), the FDA has blocked the use of needed drugs and has constituted an incredibly enormous red-tape-producing machine through which applications for new drugs must move, at terribly prohibitive costs both in terms of time and money. The result is what doctors term "the drug lag," the time between when knowledge has developed that something is good in treatment and the time it somehow becomes "legal" through FDA approval — *as if government itself, rather than science, has any right to make such an approval.*

Just how honest the FDA bureaucracy is, or how honest it *can* be vis-a-vis such vested interests as the drug trust and food processing industry, was brought into question for the umpteenth time in 1975. In the winter of that year, Congressional auditors and the General Accounting Office (GAO) found that more than 150 officials of the FDA had violated the U.S. government's own "conflict of interest" rules by owning stock in companies which the FDA regulates! (The comfortable relationship between the FDA, the AMA and drug companies was explored by Griffin in *World Without Cancer*, as well as by Beall and Josephson.)

Moreover, the GAO found that the FDA had not adequately monitored th testing of new drugs to assure the accuracy and reliability of the data on which the drugs are approved for general use. Just how honest *is* the FDA if its officers have a vested interest in major drug companies? Following the Watergate and Lockheed scandals of 1974-1976, the question is entirely fair. Then add testimony even from an FDA agent and a Congressman as to the drug industry's domination of medical education, and the question moves into sharper focus:

Chairman Gaylord Nelson of the Senate Select Committee on Small Business reported in April 1976 that "the almost complete takeover by the (drug) industry of postgraduate medical 'education' is cause for alarm." Dr. J. Richard Crout of the FDA had told the committee that the drug industry selects and pays for "the bulk of educational information provided to the practicing physician."[4]

How interested is the FDA in actually protecting consumer health? How interested is the American Cancer Society, with a $100-million-per-year take, offices, officers, overhead and budget, in actually eliminating cancer *rather than continuing to look for the answer?* How conveniently overlapped are the FDA, AMA directorate and the drug trust? These are vital questions deserving of exhaustive replies.

Small wonder that "health food fanatics," vitamin, mineral and food supplement proponents, some naturopaths, chiropractors and metabolic therapists, have all railed at the existence of a medical-industrial-governmental conspiracy, a convergence of vested interests both at the economic and political level which suppresses unwanted and rational approaches to medicine in exchange for irrational, costly and unworkable procedures.

This is strong stuff. These allegations parallel the Birch view, at least in part. The latter assessment, that medical-governmental orthodoxy is but a reflection of a graver problem, was expounded by Alan Stang in the Birch monthly magazine, *American Opinion*, in January 1974:

> *It is important not to blame doctors as a group for the underhanded campaign against Laetrile. Most doctors deserve the great respect they are paid. Rather, bureaucrats and key members of the medical establishment are responsible, and they are trying to prevent curious physicians from learning more. They are trying to keep them in line, just as the Establishment as a whole is trying to keep the American people in line.*[5]

The arrests of Drs. Richardson, Privitera and others; the "peer review" and arrest of Dr. Jones; the indictments against American and Mexican Laetrile proponents as smugglers, including wholesale violations of Constitutional rights through entrapment procedures and false statements; the enormous use of taxpayer funds in cracking down on "the Laetrile underground"; the renewed venom of the FDA in trying to eliminate apricot kernels from health-food stores; the FDA's move against Laetrile-like products through producing "doctored" evidence (see Chapter 8); the frenzy of medical orthodoxy through "establishment" journals and much of the major media to denounce Laetrile and character-assassinate its proponents — all these things only fed the conspiracy feelings of a growing segment of freedom-of-choice champions as 1976 became the tide-turning year in the battle for medical freedom.

CHAPTER FIVE

Enter John Beard

THE LAETRILE STORY BEGINS early in human history, and throughout it is studded with ironies and coincidences, the stuff that makes truth stranger than fiction. Among the more fascinating coincidences is the name of the substance itself, particularly so when compared to the name of a remedy first reported in 1813 — a kind of elixir that, among many other things, was said to cure breast cancer. The product was called Leotrill, and as far as we know it is mentioned only and exclusively in something called *The Indian Doctor's Dispensatory*, published in Cincinnati in 1813 and "being Father Smith's advice respecting diseases and their cure."[1] The author writes:

> *About thirty years ago I called on old Dr. Wilkey, a German, who had been in the business of his profession, in the Flanders wars. He proposed to me to spend a few days with him, to instruct me in some knowledge which he had gained in his long life, and which he regretted should die with him: especially to make his Leotrill, a liquid which he prepared; for the obtaining of. which he had paid a large sum in Flanders.*
>
> *With this medicine he made many of his cures, both in physic and surgery. With this, said he, "I can put a person in a complete salivation in ten minutes. I need only throw this with a syringe into any sore, ulcer, or wound, and it is fit at once for healing ... and a cancer in a woman's breast, I have never failed to cure with it."*

We will never know what went into this elixir. The Laetrile developers had never heard of this particular folk remedy, and had no notion about whether it had anything to do with Laetrile — the name Ernst Krebs, Jr. wrought out of the scientific description of his specific compound: LAEvo-mandeloniTRILE.

For the laetrilists, the natural approach to cancer must have been known in ancient China, where substances of the family of which Laetrile is really only a brand name were used medically. And, as researcher

Herbert M. Summa points out, the Egyptians in the time of the pharaohs knew the poisonous action of consuming large amounts of apricot and bitter almond kernels containing the same substance (amygdalin), of which Laetrile, again, is a brand name now in the public domain.[2]

According to Summa, the Egyptians forced people condemned to death to drink a concoction made of such kernels with water. The "apricot death," similar to a Greek process, was based on the spontaneous setting free of hydrogen cyanide from amygdalin in the intestines by the enzyme emulsin. That cyanide is a part of the amygdalin process — however perfectly natural this is in life itself — has been a specter that has haunted Laetrile from the beginning, for it has been easy for orthodoxy to concentrate on the word "cyanide" and to forget that the same cyanide-containing substances have been associated with medication. Modern research (including that of Summa) has emphasized time and time again the essential nontoxity of the purified, crystallized, extracted amygdalin called Laetrile. The referred-to Egyptian and Greek potions released "unphysiological quantities of hydrocyanic acid (which were) absolutely lethal, when liberated by enzymatic activity from a specific substrate under ideal conditions," Summa notes.

The Roman medicinal preparation called *Aqua Amygdalarum Amarum* was made from a watery emulsion of bitter almonds. This "bitter almond water" continued as a medicine known for centuries, with amygdalin supplying its source until replaced by a synthetic benzaldehyde. Bitter almonds are a primary source of amygdalin, the chemical or generic name for what later became Laetrile — a processed, purified form of the natural substance.

It is here that we should clarify some terms, since products and substances, some involving manufactured words, have been used to describe what is essentially the same thing. The name "Laetrile" (and also "laetrile") is used to refer to:

• The present injectable form of amygdalin and the extract prepared in tablet form.

• A whole class of substances in nature, scientifically and variously referred to as beta-cyanophoric glycosides, beta-cyanogenetic glucosides, and similar designations; and, more specifically, to amygdalin and prunasin, the two beta-cyanogenetic glucosides of most medical interest.

• Vitamin B-17, a designation created by Ernst T. Krebs, Jr. The McNaughton Foundation, sponsor of Laetrile research around the world, uses the designation exclusively to describe amygdalin, although Krebs broadly applies it to the beta-cyanogenetic glucosides. His term of choice for this class of substances, also coined by him, is "nitriloside."

Krebs, Jr. has defined the nitrilosides as "water-soluble, essentially non-toxic, sugary compounds found in ... plants, many of which are edible.... They comprise molecules made of a sugar, hydrogen cyanide, a benzene ring or an acetone."[3] The general designation "Laetrile" thus broadly covers amygdalin, prunasin, vitamin B-17, nitriloside, beta-cyanogenetic glucosides, beta-cyanophoric glycosides, etc. The differences mean little since all the products are essentially (but by no means specifically) the same thing when broken down in water. Amygdalin is the common chemical term occurring in the history of the substance. The latter, which is found in a wide variety of kernels and seeds, was prepared in its pure state by Pierre Jean Robiquet and Boutron in 1830. In 1837 two German scientists, Justus von Liebig and Friedrich Wohler, discovered that amygdalin is split by an enzyme complex into one molecule of hydrogen cyanide, one of benzaldehyde, and two molecules of sugar. They found the enzyme complex, with glucoside, in the bitter almond.

But the first specific use of a Laetrile-like substance in cancer that can be documented is apparently that referred to in the *Gazette Medicale de Paris* (tome XIII) of September 13, 1845, by a Dr. T. Inosemtzeff, professor of the Imperial University of Moscow.[4] In this citation, the professor described two cases of disseminated cancer apparently "controlled" successfully — one for over eleven years, the other for over three years — by the use of amygdalin. If the Paris medical journal account is indeed the first documented statement concerning cancer therapy with amygdalin, it would make 1834 the first year in which the Western world attempted to treat the crippling disease with a food factor.

But the rationale on which Ernst T. Krebs, Jr. rested a large part of his own background in the development of Laetrile or vitamin B-17, and on which a broad span of his own philosophy is based, is the relatively obscure work of a Scottish embryologist, Dr. John Beard (1858-1924), who had published his findings first in 1902 in the British journal *Lancet* and then in 1911 in the book *The Enzyme Treatment of Cancer and Its Scientific Basis*.[5] In his writings Beard elaborated a theory of the origin of cancer as novel and revolutionary (and actually simple) as any breakthrough in science. It received little more than passing interest, and some hostile commentary. To this day, his basic theory of cancer is rarely taught, little understood, and accorded not much more than a footnote of passing interest.

Beard had found himself deeply involved with the study of a cell called the trophoblast. This mysterious cell, identified in 1857 and named in 1876, was known to play a specific role in pregnancy — eating out a niche in the uterine wall where the fertilized egg could gain nutrition from the mother's bloodstream. In orthodox embryology it is regarded as a layer of extraembryonic ectoderm and its name comes from the Greek words meaning "nourishment" and "tissue."

It was the activity of the trophoblast that puzzled Beard, as it has intrigued other scientists. An invading, autonomous, erosive cell that during pregnancy may be found in the blood and other organs outside the uterus, the trophoblast behaves in ways extremely similar to cancer. It was Beard who first asked himself the spine-tingling question: Is it possible the trophoblast — a natural part of the life cycle — and the cancer cell are the same thing? He decided to find out by tracing the histories of both kinds of cells.

He worked with elasmobranchs in order to be able to study the fertilized egg many times at all its various stages. He learned that the trophoblast arises, some way, from the primitive, undifferentiated germ cell. The trophoblast creates a protective covering for the embryo (the amnion) and the nutritive organ (the chorion) through which, by absorption, the embryo receives nourishment from the mother's blood in the first weeks of pregnancy.

Beard's studies were so carefully performed that (as later noted by Krebs, Jr. and Sr. and Howard Beard — no relation to the Scottish embryologist) he was able to state that it is in the fifty-sixth day in the span of human gestation that the cellular trophoblast begins to undergo a dramatic deterioration. The time coincides with the development of the secreting function of the fetal pancreas. Something checked the further growth of the gestational trophoblast, Beard believed, and the work of these invading, eroding cells began to diminish and stop — except in one instance.

The exception is when one of the most malignant forms of cancer known, chorionepithelioma (cancer of the chorion), develops. The disease can kill a mother and child in a matter of weeks. Doctors in Beard's day conceded that trophoblasts contributed somehow to the development of chorionepithelioma, but were not certain how. Beard concerned himself with determining what it is that in effect shuts down or fails to shut down the trophoblast, hence spelling the difference between whether the fetus will live or deadly chorionepithelioma will develop.[6]

It was Beard who found the concomitance between the commencing function of the fetal pancreas and the beginning degeneration of the trophoblast. Broad comparative studies lent weight to his thesis that, in the span of normal gestation, the pancreatic enzymes are responsible for checking the growth of the gestational trophoblast, although it is not entirely destroyed. So trophoblast cells — characterized by their invasiveness, corrosiveness, erosiveness, and ability to metastasize (that is, to spread) — are normal to the life cycle and are naturally inhibited within that cycle, Beard reasoned.

Beard turned his attention to another reality about the primitive germ cells that, undergoing differentation, could ultimately be expressed as trophoblast. In the developing fetus, the majority of the primitive, undifferentiated germ cells cluster in the gonads, quite in accord with the demands of nature, since in the sex organs they mature into sperms or ova. But a minority of them (variously estimated at twenty to thirty percent) are dispersed, or "migrate," apparently at random, throughout the extragenital areas. Some of these dispersed germ cells come to rest in almost any part of the fetus and embryo. Under specific circumstances, they may attempt development into the life cycle, part of that development being the trophoblast. That is, the gross manifestation of this process outside the uterus might occur; at which time it is called *cancer*.

Moreover, Beard reasoned, if pancreatic enzymes are the inhibitors of the trophoblast in the span of gestation, then surely they should also be able to inhibit the trophoblast when it is extragenitally exhibited as cancer. If, for whatever reason, either the pancreas was not doing its job or the pancreatic enzymes were blocked in their action, then chorionepithelioma might develop — and surely, Beard reasoned, this meant that the same deficiency would also indicate that extrauterine trophoblast would also remain unchecked and would ultimately be manifested as cancer.

It has remained for researchers who took up the early work of John Beard to apply it with more data and research to the cancer riddle, to probe just what it is that stimulates the action whereby an undifferentiated germ cell may ultimately develop into trophoblast (cancer). And it is there that the massive work and research by Krebs, Jr. (though some of his conclusions are disputed by Gurchot, who also wrote on the subject) come into play.

Krebs indicates that the natural inhibition of trophoblast occurs as specific enzymes attack the "shield" of the trophoblast or neoplastic (cancer) cell, hence destroying the immunity of the trophoblast and allowing the lymphocytes to attack it. The malignant cell is also open to further digesting by the "deshielding" enzymes themselves, Krebs postulates.

In elaborating his thesis, Beard focused on the trypsins as the pancreatic enzymes that inhibit trophoblast (cancer), but emphasized that all the pancreatic enzymes were probably involved. Subsequent research has described chymotrypsin, particularly, and other enzymes as involved in the inhibitor effect.

For Beard, researching and writing seventy years ago, it all seemed to fall into place:

1. The trophoblast cell in pregnancy and the neoplastic or cancer cell

are actually one and the same thing — two manifestations (one in gestation, one outside of gestation) of the same process.

2. The trophoblast has a specific, positive role to play in pregnancy. Outside of pregnancy it is exhibited as cancer.

3. The trophoblast in pregnancy is inhibited by pancreatic enzymes; hence, the trophoblast outside of pregnancy, cancer, should be inhibited by them as well.

4. Therefore, the treatment for cancer should be pancreatic enzymes.

Beard also believed the stereochemical structure of cancer proteins and cancer carbohydrates is opposite to the structure of the same things in normal tissue.

It was the research and study of Krebs, Jr. that added more detail to the process, at least insofar as describing what might be taking place. Krebs, Jr. and Sr. and Howard Beard, along with other researchers before them, postulate in their article on the matter[7] that it is the action of the female hormone estrogen, present in both sexes, that is the trigger of the change of the undifferentiated germ cells (which the Krebs work refers to as "diploid totipotent," meaning, in essense, able to reproduce a whole new entity), "with the consequent production of a gametogenous cell whose only alternative to death is division with the resulting production of trophoblast."

In this view, based on the work of Beard and brought to the modern era, it is incorrect to call cigarette smoking, specific viruses, various chemicals, poisons, radiation, and pollution *causes* of cancer. Their actions may very well elicit estrogen, and it is estrogen that, in the presence of undifferentiated cells which might be found anywhere in normal tissue, sets off the chain of events, of which cancer is the gross exhibition. That is, they may *organize* cancer, but not *cause* it. If Krebs *et al* are correct, the only real cancer-causing agent (carcinogen) is estrogen, the innocent, natural stimulus to a chain reaction that will continue if the body's natural defenses against that reaction (pancreatic enzymes and the immunological system) are not functioning or their functions are somehow blocked.

It remained for Ernst T. Krebs, Jr. to define the pancreatic enzyme-immunological defense as the *intrinsic*, natural defense against cancer, whose deficiency would help bring cancer into being; and also to postulate that there is an *extrinsic*, natural factor in nutrition that constitutes the second line of defense against the disease.

For the researchers and scientists who argued among themselves as to details of Beard's work and the theories which might flow from them, Beard had postulated the nature — the probable cause and control — of cancer. But his work was destined to go the way of that of many other scientists. Divergent from mainstream views, it was essentially ignored.

Beard proved to be ahead of his time as far as the enzyme approach to cancer (and probably the nature of cancer itself) is concerned. It was many years before his work, declining gradually into virtual obscurity, was revived in California.

Ideas do not die. Nor did Beard's. The John Beard Memorial Foundation, established in San Francisco by the developers of what was to become Laetrile or vitamin B-17 — particularly the two Krebses and pharmacologist Dr. Charles Gurchot — was set up to perpetuate his work. It was the Beardian work on the enzymatic nature of cancer that underlies what the Krebses later called the *unitarian* or *trophoblastic thesis* of cancer. The Krebses, Dr. Gurchot, Dr. Howard Beard, and Dr. Frederick Shively have been the principals in continuing the original work of John Beard.

It should be pointed out here that by no means do all the researchers and supporters of Laetrile express complete concurrence with the John Beard thesis, or with its updating by Krebs, Jr. as the unitarian or trophoblastic thesis. Krebs, Jr., who remains an outspoken champion of Beardianism, insists this less than complete concurrence is due to the failure of medical orthodoxy to train students in the unitarian thesis. Since they are not well grounded in embryology and a series of linking disciplines, Krebs charges, young medics are graduated who have no grasp of what he sees as the true nature of the second-major killer disease in the United States.

Too, such pre-Laetrile pioneers as Dr. Gurchot, the younger Krebs' former teacher, question the validity of Beardianism to explain the entire nature of cancer. Dr. Gurchot, who also wrote on Beardianism,[8] told me that, as far as he is concerned, "the Beard theory is not completely correct. You can say Beard is *essentially* right, that he is *probably* right, but this is not so in all details."

Also, Dr. Gurchot dissents from Krebs' interpretation of the rise of the trophoblast: "The onset of cancer should be modified to say that trophoblast will result from the development of a germ cell through gametogenesis — with or without meiosis," he said, as the result of correspondence with another scientist, J. B. S. Haldane.

Dr. Gurchot speaks of totipotent (not specifically diploid totipotent) cells as dispersed through the soma or natural tissue, and believes that while estrogen indubitably plays a role, it may not be estrogen exclusively that excites the chain of events whose ultimate expression may be trophoblast (cancer). "All cancer-producing substances do have estrogenic properties," Gurchot told me. "It certainly appears that estrogen may have a good deal to do with cancer development."[9]

As early as 1944 and the "modern era" of cancer research, at least one more voice was added to the idea cancer might, conceivably, be a very natural part of the scheme of things — a suspicion later updated by Ernst T. Krebs, Jr., when he stated his belief that there is nothing naturally malignant in the universe.

Charles Oberling observed, in 1944: "Some day, perhaps, it will turn out to be one of the ironies of nature that cancer, responsible for so many deaths, still is so indissolubly connected with life."[10]

It should be stressed here that while there is at least philosophical intimacy between the evolution of Laetrile and its presumptive chemistry and Beardianism itself, not all defenders of Laetrile by any means agree that the universal answer to the question of the cause of cancer has been found within the unitarian or trophoblastic thesis. They make this statement while nonetheless supporting Laetrile as the best extant weapon against cancer.

For orthodoxy and officialdom, the theory might be said to explain the development of some specific forms of cancer, but they reject out of hand — and with painfully little enthusiasm for looking into the matter — Beardian pronouncements suggesting that the trophoblast approach explains all, or most, cancers. This, of course, springs from the conventional wisdom, still held in the 1970s, that cancer is a widely varied series of diseases, whose total causes and controls are not yet known. The epidemic incidence of cancer is the best indicator that orthodoxy and officialdom are far from the mark.

CHAPTER SIX

"My God, It Works!"

HOW THE ALMOST MIRACULOUS properties of Laetrile, or vitamin B-17, came to be known is a story of coincidences and lucky breaks, spiced by a considerable dash of hardheaded individualism.

The coincidences abound — not the least of them being that the family name of the father-son team who devoted so much of their lives to the cancer riddle, Krebs, means "cancer" in German; and that Ernst T. Krebs, Jr.'s processed vitamin B-17 was given a brand name highly reminiscent of, but utterly without any connection to, the patent medicine from the early nineteenth century mentioned earlier. That another Beard helped update the original theory of John Beard (no relation), and that the eventual use of apricot kernels as the source of Laetrile was based on a botanical classification error by the elder Krebs are other tantalizing elements.

I did not know Krebs, Sr. personally; he died months before I became interested in the vitamin B-17 story. But I met several people who knew him, including his patients, and they uniformly recalled his loving, kindly character. His early efforts to unlock the cancer riddle are the second major strand of the story. The first is the pioneering enzyme theory of John Beard.

What eventually grew out of Ernst Krebs, Sr.'s virtual obsession with bull-dogging the cause and cure of cancer was something called "the extrinsic control of cancer." That is, the use of an accessory food factor as a vital weapon against clinical cancer and, even more exciting, its probable use as *the* cancer preventative.

Born in 1877 in San Luis Obispo, California, Ernst Krebs, Sr. earned his medical degree from the College of Physicians and Surgeons, San Francisco, and then practiced in various parts of the western United States for the better part of two decades. Ernst Krebs, Jr., the first of his four children, was born in 1912 in Carson City, Nevada, where his father, a classical country doctor setting forth on his rounds on horseback or in a carriage, also worked as a physician among the Washoe Indians. (One Washoe, an orphan girl, was adopted into the Krebs family.)

Some of the early remembrances of Krebs, Sr. come from Dr. Charles Gurchot, a pharmacologist who worked with him for years in pursuit of the enzymatic control of cancer. It was Gurchot, along with Dr. Leon Lewis, who was a stimulus for the elder Krebs to persevere in the development of his special compound. Dr. Gurchot told me of the strange and at times amusing events that led Krebs Sr. into the cancer problem, and his son into developing what came to be Laetrile.

Krebs, Sr., though a physician, had also studied pharmacy. He had a marked flair for investigation, research, and new ideas — traits that would also become apparent in his son. He set up his own laboratory in San Francisco's Mission District and maintained his office above a pharmacy across the street. The Krebs family settled into a Queen Anne mansion on South Van Ness Avenue. In this stately edifice both Krebses lived, studied, and worked. Krebs, Sr., still active in his nineties, was a fixture at the home until his last day. Krebs, Jr. maintains his office there today.

When the elder Krebs turned his attention to the development of new ideas in medicine, he incurred his first negative brushes with medical orthodoxy — particularly when he produced an antibiotic called Balsamea to aid in the treatment of respiratory ailments. Though this occurred ten years before Sir Alexander Fleming discovered penicillin in 1928, all Krebs, Sr. received was criticism. Told by the American Medical Association that Balsamea was worthless, he withdrew from the medical association and never rejoined.

More than Balsamea came out of Krebs's Balsamea Laboratory, though, and he became known as an innovative, experimenting physician. How these innovations and experiments ultimately turned to the apricot has been recalled in detail by Dr. Gurchot, who was told the whole story by Krebs, Sr. himself.

"During Prohibition, whiskey was smuggled into San Francisco from boats," Gurchot remembered. "The smuggled stuff sometimes had wood alcohol in it, so the smugglers had their stuff analyzed for wood alcohol before anyone bought it. To do this, they had to give it to a lab. So it wasn't strange that he (Krebs) got a great many calls from bootleggers to see if he could analyze their alcohol.

"At first, he said he was not equipped to do this, but he got so many calls he figured it would be lucrative to get into the alcohol analysis business. So he finally accepted, and started analyzing specimens. He said most of the stuff was awful and tasted terrible, and he wondered why somebody couldn't make a synthetic bourbon flavor and add alcohol to it. So he set himself to this problem and got a dentist to work with him."

Gurchot remembers that Krebs, Sr. told him he was particularly interested in determining what role the aging process played in changing the taste of the whisky and also how the various impure ingredients, which often caused consumers to become ill, could be cleansed from the product. Gradually he focused his attention on the staves of the oak barrels containing the smuggled whiskey, particularly in cases where the alcohol content was sufficiently low and the water content sufficiently high to allow the growth of a kind of mold, which Krebs called "cryptogams" (after the old name for plants not having true flowers and seeds).

The probing physician determined that the mold produced enzymes, which were released into the alcohol and worked on the raw whiskey. But only a very small amount of the mold was available, producing a very small amount of enzyme; this caused the aging process — faithful to its name — to take a long time.

His curiosity piqued as to what kind of enzymes were present in the barrel staves, Dr. Krebs next made shavings from the oak staves, Dr. Gurchot recalled, and moistened them with the nutrients that might be derived from the whiskey. He added vitamins and flour made from acorns, "which he decided was a very good nutrient." The shavings were toasted to a golden brown, moistened with water containing vitamin B-1 and acorn flour, and this mixture was ground up in water. Krebs let the preparation stand in a glass-covered jar for a few days. At the end of this time, Krebs discovered the concoction to be covered by a hairlike growth of mold.

He next poured the raw whiskey over the mold preparation on the oak and allowed it to remain for several days. He then removed the raw whiskey, filtered it, and boiled the resulting product. After thirty days the process had "remarkably" changed the taste of the whiskey. Still determined to find out what enzymes were involved, he learned that proteolytic (that is, protein-digesting) enzymes played a role when he put up a liquid extract of the mixture with the white of an egg and left it overnight. The substance ate the egg white. "This was the cataclysmic event," Dr. Gurchot recalled. "Dr. Krebs told me, 'When I saw that enzyme doing all that digesting, it occurred to me it could be useful in cancer. Maybe you think I'm crazy, but that's what I thought. The idea haunted me, so I decided to try and find out if it could do anything good in cancer.'"

It did indeed become an obsession. Plunging into the work that had originally been stimulated by the hunt to determine how the taste of smuggled whiskey could be improved, Krebs began trapping rats in the basement of his home, hoping to catch one with a tumor so he could see if his oak mold extract might have a similar effect — that is, if it would "digest" the tumor. This series of events all occurred in the early 1920s. Finally, the senior Krebs did find rats with tumors. He thought they were cancerous but did not conduct laboratory tests. He started a series of injections and these early tests did in fact indicate some ability in regressing tumors. The fact that some treated rats remained frisky and ran away indicated to him that the injected substance was essentially nontoxic; but at least one rat died. The results, then, were scattered and the conditions were hardly scientific. But Krebs was sure he definitely was on to something.

At some point during the experiments his initial batch of material ran out, and when he prepared a second supply it was not effective. He made a third supply of extract with the same lack of results and even ordered "bourbon oak" from Kentucky. There was no success with this, either. What to do? Anyone else would have given up, but not Dr. Krebs. His thinking, recalled Gurchot, was that "perhaps if I use some other plant that is related I can get an extract that is not capricious." Gurchot recalled: "He said to me, 'the oak belongs to the rose family — therefore, if I could use the extract of a plant from the rose family maybe it could be active.'" The error, noted Gurchot, is that the oak does *not* belong to the rose family. But no matter, Krebs kept a look-out for plants he presumed to be from that family.

It is here that a family interest played a key role. The Washoe Indian girl invited into the family earlier had grown up, fallen in love with a young Hawaiian, and married him. Gurchot said he recalled that the young man was related to the last queen of the Hawaiian Islands, Liliuokalani (1838-1917). The Washoe-Hawaiian couple received a $50,-000 inheritance. With it, they moved to Oakland, California, and bought a ranch of apricot trees.

"They kept relations with the Krebs family," Gurchot said. "Apricots belong to the rose family, so Krebs thought he would have a ready supply, figuring the extracts could be obtained from the seeds and kernels. So he made an extract and, lo and behold, it *was* effective." The process, Gurchot continued, consisted of removing the oil from the kernels, grinding them up in water, filtering the soup, precipitating the filtrate with alcohol, drying the precipitate, redissolving it, then injecting it. There is at this point some confusion as to exactly how much animal experimentation went on, and exactly when the extract was first used experimentally on humans.

Wynn Westover, a staff consultant to the McNaughton Foundation, has done much of the research on the early Krebs papers that refer to the development and use of this early extract, and he has noted that the physician believed he was extracting enzyme substances from the apricot kernel. "Among the substances he tentatively identified were 'emulsin, amygdalase, prunase, pectinase, and others," Westover wrote.[1]

Glenn Kittler records that some of Krebs' tests involved work with mice especially bred to respond readily to the various carcinogens known to elicit cancer.[2] Such animals could even be purchased with cancers growing in specified areas. These tests, again, showed mixed results: There were reductions in some tumors, but other mice died — some quite suddenly. That there was some effect from the extract seemed obvious, but that it had some toxicity also seemed obvious. Gurchot said he did not recall Krebs ever mentioning the precise events as mentioned by Kittler, adding that the physician found the extract mostly nontoxic.

The pharmacologist remembered that when Krebs finally turned to the use of his presumably harmless extract on humans, he found a relatively consistent pattern of pain reduction and other mixed, but generally optimistic, results. There are divergent accounts of just how and when he turned to work on humans. But eventually he did, and he continued to work on trying to purify and improve the extract. The investigative doctor pursuing the elusive answer to cancer did not charge his cancer patients, and his research with them eventually cut into his regular medical practice, but by then the cancer battle had become his primary preoccupation.

Gurchot recalled that of about twenty-five of the early cases he had discussed with Krebs, there were no toxic effects *per se*, even though cancer-stricken patients reported some side effects, usually chills and illusions like "crawling of ants" in the tumor area. But cancer patients across the board reported the reduction or complete disappearance of pain — a dramatic analgesic effect.

About the year 1928 or 1929 the first patients were injected with the new extract which Dr. Krebs had previously tested on animals, Westover reports. It was a little later than this that Gurchot met Dr. Krebs. This was because both he and medical doctor Leon Lewis were working at Sonoma State Home, a California state hospital, and were involved in research on enzymes and cancer. When they learned that a San Francisco Mission District doctor was also experimenting with enzyme chemistry and cancer, they became interested and got together with him, thus touching off a collaboration that was to last for many years.

By this time, Gurchot remembered, the senior Krebs, who had become intensely interested in enzymes and was reading all he could about them, had elaborated a theory of the beta-glucosidic structure of cancer protein, "because cancer was apparently successfully treated by a beta-glucosidic enzyme, emulsin." This was basically the theory Krebs was working on at the outset of the investigative collaboration, beginning in 1932, with Doctors Gurchot (a pharmacologist and biochemist) and Lewis (an M.D.). The collaboration, Gurchot insists, served to revitalize the senior Krebs' interest because the San Francisco physician had become "disgusted" with the derisive attention his enzyme approach had received.

Krebs made available to them several ampuls of his extract and Lewis tried it on a cancer patient. The result of the first use by Lewis, Gurchot recalled, caused the physician to exclaim, "My God, it works!" Under appropriate conditions, it was determined that the patient was showing several changes, particularly reduction in pain. This first case revealed an enormous potential for further research.

Since Krebs, Sr. believed emulsin was the essential cancer-combating ingredient in the extract, Gurchot prepared a batch of extract with the enzymes killed. "I didn't tell him (Krebs)," he said. "Then a few weeks later I asked him to see how active the material was. He reported he had treated people successfully. I told him it didn't have any emulsin in it and at first he didn't believe me." The three scientists continued trying to find what the active ingredient was. Gurchot recalled that the mystery of the active ingredient was not solved until well into the 1940s. But for the time being, he knew that something in the extract was having a definite positive effect on cancer patients.

As a result of correspondence with Krebs in 1933 the International Cancer Research Foundation in Philadelphia invited Gurchot and Lewis to the Eastern city for a year, with full cooperation promised for clinical (human) studies of the Krebs extract. The clinical studies were conducted in three large hospitals, and research on the presumed enzymes was carried out at Cornell University in Ithaca, New York, with Gurchot in charge. Lewis and Gurchot were told that they would be given only very advanced cases because "all we want to do is see if there is any change taking place at all." At the end of a year, the results were to be assessed to see what the next course of action should be.

Gurchot remembered that for a year the "moribund" human cancer cases were treated by injection. Effects were noted strongly indicative of positive palliation — even tumor size reduction, though the patients ultimately died. Gurchot recalled with amazement that "during all this time nobody (from the medical staffs) even came to observe — but nobody." So when the year was up and all the Californians had to show for their efforts was a list of dead cancer victims, they were told the project would not be continued. And the man who was to become Ernst T. Krebs, Jr.'s mentor returned to California to teach at the University of California Medical School's Department of Pharmacology. Gurchot continued his interest in the cancer problem, never losing his belief that the Krebs extract had an obvious key role to play in its solution.

In the meantime, the Krebs extract had received attention elsewhere. Wynn Westover of the McNaughton Foundation, rummaging around in the Krebs attic, found and collated many of the documents and correspondence relating to the use by other scientists of that extract in the 1930s. Among them are references to a Tokyo physician named Hatta using enzyme cancer treatments, one of which involved saving "an inoperable breast and gland involvement case in the royal family." Another, from patent attorney T. Akiyama, suggests that the seed of *Prunus armeniaca* (apricot) was "known to the public from old times . . . internally or externally applied as a medicine for tumors." Notations and correspondence from China, Czechoslovakia, Canada, and Austria indicated treatments with or clinical trials of enzyme extracts, aside from the cases being studied in the United States.

In 1934 and 1935 Dr. Krebs also collaborated with Dr. Arthur Stoll of Basel, Switzerland; each sent the other ampuls of extract prepared according to the Krebs formula and each continued clinically testing the products of the other. About the same results were obtained in both countries: regression of tumors and relief of pain. From then through 1938, several physicians around the world were experimenting with the Krebs extract, including New York City's Dr. James Ewing, who became a steadfast supporter of the formula and its need for much wider testing in human cancer cases.

This was the atmosphere in which Ernst Krebs, Jr. grew up — cleaning up after laboratory animals, taking care of supplies, and acquiring the painstaking attention to detail necessary for the empirical method and the hours of experiments and testing he would later carry out. The intellectual atmosphere was also stimulating, for science, religion, philosophy, and art were regular concerns at the Krebs mansion. Krebs, Jr. became a philosopher of sorts; his mind reached out to understand the mechanics of health and disease in an orderly universe.

The junior Krebs, reportedly a brilliant student in school, decided to follow in his father's footsteps and entered Hahnemann Medical College in Philadelphia. Eventually he attended the University of Illinois and received his bachelor's degree in bacteriology; he then transferred to the University of California for matriculation in pharmacology and, later, in anatomy. The fact that Krebs, Jr.'s doctorate degree is honorary rather than "earned" has been used by opponents of Laetrile to pillory him in print. However, the Krebs studies in a wide variety of fields, and backed by what Krebs, Jr. describes as some two dozen patents for his medical and scientific work, and by several hundred citations in medical and scientific literature, should be more than enough to give him every ounce of scientific credentialing necessary for acceptance among peers.

It was during the summer of 1938 that the young medical student went to work for Dr. Gurchot in the latter's pharmacological laboratory at the University of California. At this time, Gurchot was investigating any and all explanations for the origin and treatment of cancer, a pursuit which paralleled the younger Krebs' growing interest in the enzyme approach his father and Gurchot were continuing to work on. During the younger Krebs' visits to the Gurchot laboratory, during vacation periods and other times, he expressed an interest in becoming a graduate student in pharmacology to work on the problem. He did indeed matriculate as a pharmacology student and thus began the second collaboration under Gurchot, sometimes stormy, which would finally lead to Laetrile.

At this point, none of the principals knew about the John Beard theory; they were simply pursuing the enzyme approach to cancer treatment. Gurchot and Krebs, Jr. and other students talked about "curious methods of treating cancer that had been used," said Gurchot. "So one day in 1938 Krebs burst in carrying a book, slapped it down and said, 'Here's one for your collection.'" Young Krebs, an avid reader, had become attracted to the old tome because of the word "enzyme" in its title. It was, in fact, John Beard's 1911 book, *The Enzyme Treatment of Cancer*.

Gurchot recalls that he simply placed it on his microscope table and didn't begin to peruse it until a couple of weeks later. "The more I read it, the more amazed I became," he said. His own wide background in various linking disciplines convinced him of Beard's "remarkable biology." After immersing himself in Beard's work (first published in 1902), "I realized the guy really had worked out the cause, the biology of cancer," Gurchot recalled. "I gave a seminar on it. Everybody was fascinated. I gave three lectures on it at the UC Medical School. After it was all over, the doctors thought it was the greatest thing ever — or the greatest hoax. So I read more about Beard."

When Krebs, Jr. returned from a vacation, the two men, mentor and student, discussed the work. There are diverging accounts of what happened next, but the result is that young Krebs, the voracious reader, decided to check out the Beard theory as far as he could through intensive reading and research. The spark was ignited that would fire Krebs, Jr.'s own obsession, which would lead not only to the discovery of Laetrile but to the entire vitamin B-17 concept of cancer prevention. The challenge of Beard caused Krebs Jr. to make a key decision: He switched from medicine to biochemistry, so he could devote full time to the cancer riddle. The young Krebs spent a total of nine years in university studies (including bacteriology, physiology, anatomy, pharmacology, and medicine). He taught himself to read French, German, Spanish, and Italian in order to peruse, over the course of years of research, over 17,000 scientific papers, books, and research documents in those languages.

The Krebs Sr.-Krebs Jr.-Gurchot collaboration focused on chymo-trypsin, one of the pancreatic enzymes that (based on the Beard theory) manifests antithesis to the trophoblast cell — which is cancer. Krebs, Jr. told me that in 1943 they developed the first crystalline chymotrypsin commercially available in the world. "It was made to be used clinically for its possibly palliative effect in human cancer," he said, noting that "the seed preparation — the apricot extract preparation — had been set aside because of its overt toxicity."

The work with chymotrypsin, proceeding on different fronts (Gurchot, from Chicago, noted fifty to sixty cases of chymotrypsin use on cancer, only one of which resulted in complete recovery), was only part of Ernst T. Krebs, Jr.'s full-time involvement. He determined to update the Beardian theory, to demonstrate that it *was* the proper explanation for the myriad manifestations of cancer and that treatment based on its premises held out the only real hope to solve the cancer problem.

After years of research, study, duplications of experiments, and appli-cations of the Euclidean principle that two things equal to the same thing are equal to each other, Krebs was ready, in 1947, to announce to the scientific world the results of his studies. His paper included a compila-tion of thirty characteristics shared by the trophoblast cell and the cancer cell, and noted the specific antithesis of chymotrypsin to cancer cells. What little attention this compilation received was mostly favorable.

But it was not until 1950 that the two Krebses, along with Texas biochemist Howard Beard, published "The 'Unitarian or Trophoblastic Thesis' of Cancer" in the *Medical Record*. This study, along with John Beard's writings a half century earlier, constitute the bible of the vitamin B-17 movement. In it, forty-two shared trophoblast (cancer) traits are noted. The medical world, strongly influenced by the viral theory of cancer — an approach dominating cancer research into the seventies — paid little attention to the paper. But the Krebses plunged on anyway, with Krebs, Jr. continuing extract experiments.

The younger Krebs had earlier found that chymotrypsin experi-ments were more discouraging than encouraging. Working apart, Gurchot (who had left the University of California in 1945 and had also ended his close collaboration with the Krebses, although the scientists remained in touch ever after) found that the sequence of events in chymotrypsin therapy seemed to go as follows: first, an immediate improvement in cancer patients, followed by a return of their symptoms. Gurchot none-theless maintained interest in Beard and in 1949 wrote *Biology — The Key to the Riddle of Cancer*.

Krebs consistently noted that chymotrypsin lacked the force to do the specific job that Beard had attributed to it in his theory. Whether other enzymes were involved or some other, missing ingredient played a role, the junior Krebs did not know. He turned to his father's earlier extract, the use of which had been complicated by the continuing presence of an unknown factor causing apparently toxic reactions. Two key elements were still puzzling about the extract: Exactly *what* did the demonstrated job of causing tumor reduction and analgesic effects? And exactly *what* caused the toxic symptoms? Krebs set out to improve the apricot-kernel preparation.

Both Gurchot and Krebs agreed that the clue to the toxicity factor was provided by former UCLA pathologist Dr. Clifford Bartlett, who demonstrated that the various reactions reported by some patients injected with the extract were the typical reactions of cyanide. The bells were now ringing in the minds of both men. Ernst Krebs recalled that the old extract did indeed contain cyanide, from the compound amygdalin (a beta-cyanogenetic glucoside that Krebs would later call vitamin B-17). The extract included a whole host of other elements and enzymes, including emulsin. Krebs toyed with the fresh and tantalizing theory that cyanide could very well be the blessing and the curse of the old extract — that selective release of cyanide at a tumor site was actually the weapon that inhibited tumors, but the premature release of the poison (for example, by the enzyme action of emulsin during the processing of the extract) would produce some toxic effects.

The theory on which the biochemist ultimately worked, and which has been a source of some controversy among the laetrilists, is this: The enzymes called beta-glycosidases, able to break down the old extract and release its cyanide, are massively present in cancerous areas. Yet, since people normally consume small amounts of cyanide daily in certain fruits and vegetables, Krebs wondered why cyanide did not destroy normal cells. He researched the properties of yet another enzyme: rhodanese. Discovered in 1933, the substance had been shown to be equipped to detoxify cyanide-bearing substances. And most important, according to Krebs, Jr.'s research, it was known that cancer cells are deficient in rhodanese. If rhodanese was a natural defense of normal tissue against cyanide, and if cancer cells were deficient in rhodanese, and if beta-glycosidase released cyanide, then quite possibly cancer was defenseless against cyanide.

Krebs set about the challenge of altering his father's extract so that the cyanide would remain safely bound in its compound until reaching the hydrolyzing (breaking-up) enzymes at cancer growth sites. In layman's terms, he had to devise a chemical pistol that would fire its fatal bullet only at the enemy. The research on amygdalin convinced him that the key lay in further refining the extract until what resulted was purified amygdalin. The process is not mysterious, he pointed out in 1974 when he addressed the San Francisco Vegetarian Society for Health and Humanity:

The first step in the present production, which is from natural materials, is to grind the apricot seed or kernel; then it is defatted with a cold solvent, such as ether, hexachlorine, or other such substance, and then the solvent is driven from the remaining ground pulp and a complete fat-free powder which is partially soluble in water is left. The Laetrile (amygdalin) in this powder as well as the sugars are also soluble in alcohol and Laetrile (amygdalin) happens to be selectively soluble in boiling alcohol about 40 times greater than in cold alcohol. The fat-free powder is then added to boiling alcohol about 40 times greater than in cold alcohol.

The fat-free powder is then added to boiling alcohol where Laetrile (amygdalin) is extracted from the powder and then the materials are filtered. The filtrate that remains is put in a freezing cabinet or refrigerator and cold room where the temperature is brought down to about 10 degrees Centigrade.

The crystals of Laetrile precipitate or fall to the bottom of the flask because in cold alcohol the material is insoluble. Now these crystals are recovered and the process of recrystallization is repeated a number of times depending upon whether the material is to be used for oral purposes or for injection.

When the chemicals are dried the first time, they have a chemical purity of about 99.7 or 99.8 percent pure. For oral purposes, it is repeated twice.[3]

Krebs, Jr. projected the possible development of synthetic forms of the extract, and his description of the chemistry in such a development excited controversy almost immediately. He derived the name "Laetrile" from a compound which he described as laevo (left-moving)-mandelonitrile-beta-glucuronoside. In earlier papers, Krebs discussed the projected or assumed actions of both the natural and the synthetic "laetriles," the key point being his assertion that specific enzymes break down specific versions of the compound.

The name "Laetrile," so close to the sound produced by "Leotrill," the patent medicine, is only one symbol of a process having come full circle. Through trial and error, hit and miss, the Krebses and their collaborators had actually *returned* to the ancient use of amygdalin in natural foods. But equipped with modern processing techniques, they were now able to process, purify, crystallize, and freeze-dry amygdalin for medical use. An intriguing chain of events had occurred:

• John Beard had postulated that the trophoblast in pregnancy and cancer are actually one and the same thing, and that a pancreatic enzyme inhibits both.

- Non-Beardian cancer researchers had become interested in enzymes as they might relate to cancer.
- An innovative, investigative M.D. with pharmaceutical training had become interested in enzymes in order to measure the effects of the aging process on bootleg whiskey. In the process, he discovered that enzymes in a whiskey-testing concoction he had made digested the white of an egg, and he then wondered if this could not somehow relate to cancer.
- By misclassifying the trees from which the whiskey barrel wood came, and through a family relationship that resulted in handy access to a supply of apricots, the same doctor was provided with the supply of a substance from which to make an extract for investigation.
- His son, piqued by curiosity, came across John Beard's book and, through him, it came into the hands of an enzyme researcher uniquely qualified to understand its full implications.
- The coordinated effort to substantiate John Beard's ideas through use of chymotrypsin was only partially successful, so the son went back to an investigation of his father's earlier extract process.
- The result of this amazing chain of developments was Laetrile.

It was not until 1949 that Ernst T. Krebs, Jr. was ready to inject himself with the first shot of the purified substance to be given to a human. While some have attempted to enshrine that moment as an instant of great danger (since theoretically cyanide was present, although the bodily defense against cyanide by rhodanese was known), Krebs shrugs off any idea of danger: "Hell, no, I wasn't scared. The odds were overwhelmingly with me. I was dealing with the known."

At any rate, he survived the first injection, he was convinced that his long years of study and work were correct in every aspect: the material was safe for human use. Had he had cancer, the enzymes would have triggered the lethal release of cyanide at the site of the tumor, while his natural noncancerous tissue was protected by rhodanese. If he had no cancer, the body's natural processes would eliminate the Laetrile naturally.

It is essential to point out here that there is not a unanimity of opinion as to the precise action of Laetrile. To this day, Dr. Charles Gurchot questions the exact series of events in the Laetrile reaction as described by Krebs and states that the cyanide action is "not proven." He told me: "It is reasonable to suppose that the action of Laetrile on cancer cells is that it releases cyanide, but this is still not conclusively proven." And Dr. Dean Burk, Laetrile's chief defender within the otherwise hostile National Cancer Institute, told me: "Both Dr. (Hans) Nieper and I have conceived of several mechanisms of action of amygdalin which have nothing to do with any action of cyanide."[4]

Part of officialdom's hostile reaction against Laetrile was based on the alleged failure of tests to duplicate the precise action described by Krebs.[5] These failings, however, fade alongside the greater achievement: Laetrile *works*! (By "works" we mean reactions varying from relief of pain, the most common reaction, to complete regression of tumors.) If it is ultimately determined that other actions are somehow involved in the process, it will constitute another example, as occurs so often in history, that Laetrile may be "right for the wrong reason."

One of the most exhaustive studies of how Laetrile may work was produced by a University of California-San Diego medical student in November 1975. Mark McCarty, who researched in detail the Laetrile controversy and the vast amount of contradiction concerning it, approached the issue with cold objectivity. He found the arguments of the anti-Laetrile forces far more wanting than those of its proponents.

Disputing, as have many, the Krebs "local release" theory, McCarty posits that amygdalin may work by producing a serum cyanide, one which does cause selective toxicity to cancer cells without impairing "host functioning," and that the mechanism involves the acidification of cancer tissue and the decreasing of glucose availability to tumor regions with poor links to the circulatory system. Cyanide-activated acidification should trigger the immune system into "surveillance" to help slow, stop or reverse tumor growth, he wrote in a splendidly researched article in a student publication.[6] McCarty's research tended to explain why Laetrile is apparently most effective against small tumors and metastases and why in test-tube experiments tumors do not seem to be selectively sensitive to cyanide, while tumors in *in vivo* do show such sensitivity.

In April 1976, A. Keith Brewer and Richard A. Passwater wrote in *American Laboratory*[7] that the presence of hydrogen cyanide and an adequate level of potassium may explain how to reverse a cancer process within cells. The cause of cancer and its answer, they suggest, may be as follows:

The attachment of cancer-causing agents (carcinogens) to cell membranes eliminates the transport of oxygen across the membranes. A drop in the hydrogen ion concentration (pH) level from 7.35 to 6 follows, due to the conversion of glucose into lactic acid as a consequence of the elimination of oxygen. Lysosomal enzymes are liberated and nucleic and amino acids are fermented within the cell as a consequence of the foregoing. The reaction of lactic acid and lysosomal enzymes with cell DNA to destroy the normal DNA-RNA (genetic) reactions and control mechanism of the cell follows. This seems to coincide with Dr. Charles Gurchot's updated Beardian theory, in which Dr. Krebs' mentor notes that trophoblast may arise from "normal tissue" if the repressed "asexual generation" genes within a normal or somatic cell are abnormally activated.

Brewer and Passwater suggest as a "possible therapy" finding the means to raise the pH to the 9 level, and add that "theoretically this could be accomplished by first feeding the animal having a low pH tumor a suitable type of nitrile which will hydrolyze in an acid medium to liberate HCN (hydrogen cyanide) within the cell" — and possibly followed by administration of cesium or rhubidium salts, which, along with potassium, constitute cell membrane "transportation" carriers of oxygen. The presence of hydrogen cyanide (HCN) within the cell membrane renders it "very pervious" to potassium, cesium and rhubidium ions, they point out. The concentration of the latter in cancer cells where HCN is present should raise the pH to the 9 level. This action should halt the proliferation of cancerous activity, allowing toxic enzymes in the inner layers of cells in a tumor to bring about the death of the cancer once proliferation has stopped.

Here, HCN — as conceivably released by amygdalin — would be serving as a catalyst for chemical activity which could retard cancer rather than being involved in a direct attack on cancer itself.

In the September 1975 issue of *Cancer Research*, a paper by Lea, Koch and Morris[8] reveals that sodium cyanate at a dose level of 125 or 250 milligrams per kilogram of body weight produced greater than 85 percent inhibition in the synthesis of protein in liver and kidney cancers in mice, with virtually no effect on normal tissues. Since proteins are the building material of cells and tissues, such an inhibition of protein is tantamount to an inhibition of greater than 85 percent in the growth of such cells and tissues. Cyanates are breakdown products of such compounds as amygdalin or any Laetrile-like substance.

The above illustrations focus on the role of hydrogen cyanide and/or cyanates as they may be variously involved in the chemistry of cancer. Whether the HCN attack on cancer in all its forms is direct or indirect; whether in some cases it is involved in a local breakdown by enzymes or is generally surveillant as serum cyanide; and whether the specific action is more involved with protein synthesis, the fact is that vitamin B-17 or Laetrile or similar substances are being vindicated as cancer fighters — even when the researchers involved never heard of Laetrile or the Krebs theory.

In the meantime, vitamin B-17 researchers have continued the hunt for uses of other beta-cyanogenetic glucosides, and it has been Ernst T. Krebs, Jr. who has propounded the theory that the full range of these substances, lumped together as vitamin B-17, constitutes the natural, extrinsic prevention of cancer when the natural, intrinsic mechanism (pancreatic enzymes and the immunological system) is malfunctioning.

For the San Francisco biochemist, an important piece of evidence in his own philosophy is being demonstrated in the cancer battle: there is nothing naturally malignant in the universe. Cancer is not formed by an alien, outside force, but through natural processes that run wild when man's tampering with nature has removed or diminished the natural restraints on those processes. In the case of cancer, the cancer cells (as trophoblast) have a specific job to do, and are a natural part of the life cycle. When they remain unchecked because the metabolism is out of balance, the result is described as cancer. Correct the metabolism, and the cancer will be inhibited — this is the chief argument of vitamin B-17 proponents.

Krebs has continued to experiment with several forms of the new, purified extract. In 1965, a study conducted for the California State Department of Public Health on the composition and chemical behavior of two kinds of Laetrile from the United States and Canada found the products minimally different from each other. One product tested contained sucrose and di-isopropyl ammonium iodide and was described as an "amorphous solid." Another, called a "colorless solution," had a trace of phenol but neither of the two other elements. In both cases, the primary ingredient was identified as amygdalin.

In its rulings against Laetrile the State of California referred specifically to the beta-cyanogentic glucosides (or "laetriles," the quotation marks added by the statutes) as the substances held to be illegal in cancer use, and specifically ruled against the two beta-cyanogenetic glucosides amygdalin (with or without di-isopropyl ammonium iodide) and prunasin, "commonly known as 'laetriles.'" In later federal tests, Laetrile was referred to as "amygdalin-MF" (McNaughton Foundation). Hence the confusion between the various descriptions: those occurring in science as amygdalin, beta-cyanogenetic glucosides, cyanophoric glucosides (and glycosides), and the Krebs-compounded words "Laetrile," "nitriloside," and "vitamin B-17" all mean essentially the same thing.

Back in 1950, proof that a cyanide-bearing compound was safe for use on humans did not mean that it was of any use in conquering cancer, so the Krebses, father and son, embarked on careful research and experimentation to build a case for the credibility of Laetrile therapy. The first Laetrile treatment of human cancers, given intramuscularly and involving only ten milligrams,' a fraction of many doses given today, was provided for the elder Dr. Krebs's terminal patients. A very small dose was used because the amount of cyanide humans could tolerate was not known. A decrease in pain was the first common reaction to those early tests on patients. Weight gain and appetite improvement were noted, too, though death still occurred. In several cases, the patient's demise was prolonged far beyond original estimates.

From the beginning, father and son ran into considerable disbelief and unwillingness to experiment with amygdalin on the part of other men in the medical profession, even when they were able to demonstrate reduction of pain and an increase in the feeling of well-being among their patients.

An early pioneer in the field was Los Angeles physician Arthur T. Harris, a South African who had been in the United States since 1928 and who was preparing to return to his homeland when he heard about the Krebses' compound. And here occurred another coincidence in the vitamin B-17 story, for Dr. Harris had studied embryology under John Beard at the University of Edinburgh, Scotland, and was fully acquainted with the long-ignored trophoblastic theory of his former mentor.

Believing that the Krebses cases and Laetrile were the proof in the pudding of Beard's theory, Dr. Harris reversed his decision to return to South Africa, opened an office in California, and, in 1951, began treating patients with the compound. His first patient was a thirty-six-year-old divorcee with cancer of the cervix who had refused treatment by surgery or radiation. The spectacular turnaround in her case — Dr. Harris reported her alive and free of cancer symptoms ten years later — encouraged treatments of other cancer patients.

In a sixteen-month period, Dr. Harris treated eighty-two patients. Three of them are clinically free of cancer today, twenty-four are still alive and comfortable, and fifty-five received only temporary help from Laetrile.

In the meantime, several other Los Angeles doctors and a New Jersey group had begun using the substance, and it was being investigated in England, Belgium, Italy, the Philippines, and Japan. Early results seemed to show Laetrile that dosages as large as 400 milligrams had no harmful effects; it was learned that intravenous injections brought better reactions than intramuscular ones did.

There were, then, several doctors actively using Laetrile in the United States. Efforts to secure grants from philanthropic institutions to pay for the Laetrile failed utterly, so most of the doctors agreed to pay for production of their supplies. They also agreed to keep their work on the compound quiet since so much more needed to be known about it.

The expression "My God, it works!" — first uttered twenty years ago — was echoed many more times around the world. There was enthusiasm among the Krebses, their collaborators, and innovative doctors in the United States. Not only had the riddle of the cause of cancer been solved, they believed, but the weapon to combat cancer had been discovered and sharpened for use. They were ready to do battle against the Big C. But the clampdown on the new hope for cancer was not long in coming.

CHAPTER SEVEN

Officialdom's Response: Crackdown on Laetrile

THE EVER-RECURRING "ORTHODOX" ATTACK on Laetrile first began in November 1952 in Santa Monica, where Dr. Harris had invited the chairman of the California Cancer Commission to take a look at Laetrile patients. As Glenn Kittler recorded in *Laetrile — Control for Cancer*, the patients were not thoroughly examined and, worse, the opinion was expressed that patients benefiting from the treatment either (a) never had cancer in the first place, (b) were responding belatedly to orthodox surgical or radiation treatment (or both), or (c), were undergoing "spontaneous remission" or "regression" of symptoms.

These three arguments persist throughout the legal battle of Laetrile as it has collided with the mind of orthodoxy: it just *could not* work, so therefore any examples of its seeming effectiveness *must* come from some other reason. Several doctors and officials told me this persistently during my own investigation, most of them being careful to add that they were not directly or entirely excluding the possibility of some Laetrile efficacy.

The terms "spontaneous remission" and "regression" are, after all, what the "counterculture" calls a "copout" — phrases suggesting that something has happened that no one understands.

It was not until March 23, 1953, that the California Cancer Commission, a department of the California Medical Association, held a press conference to announce that a "thorough" investigation of Laetrile had been made and that the compound was worthless. The "famous 44" — the cases the commission claimed to have investigated — set the primary basis for all subsequent orthodox arguments against the Krebs compound. In fact, that report was still cited by state public health department authorities as late as Summer 1976 as the best argument against Laetrile. But, as the national Cancer Institute's cytochemistry chief pointed out: "The 1953 report of the California Cancer Commission ... described no patient ever receiving a total dosage of Laetrile as great as is now the current standard *daily* dosage (3 gram/day or more)."[1]

The official conclusions of the California study read, in part: "The Commission has collected information concerning 44 patients treated with Laetrile, all of whom either have active disease or are dead of their disease, with one exception. Of those alive with disease, no patient has been found with objective evidence of control of cancer under treatment with Laetriles alone."[2] The way the last sentence reads to a layman, it could be inverted to suggest that "some patients have been found with objective control of cancer under various treatments, including Laetriles." This is a gratuitous interpretation, of course, but the semantics of the statement lead to some suggestive questions.

The report is of great importance in the Laetrile controversy because it is the major foundation on which the subsequent anti-Laetrile decisions rest. First, as the Freedom Newspapers found when they did the first, serious, in-depth study of the Laetrile phenomena in 1964, the nine physicians who formed the committee that ruled against the substance had no personal experience with Laetrile. Of the five surgeons, two radiologists, one pathologist, and one professor of medicine, not one had personal experience with the use of Laetrile.

It was not until ten years after the first report was issued that more detailed information became available. Among the data: five patients had received only one injection, five had received only two.[3] The largest amount of Laetrile listed for any patient included in the 1953 report was 2 grams, 275 milligrams in twelve injections from September 26, 1952, to December 15, 1952.

The Freedom Newspapers probe noted, moreover, that the committee's initial study reports that a biochemist to whom Laetrile samples were submitted had found in an "inconclusive study" that he was unable to break down the material to release cyanide and that the results of the tests thus "do not support the claims made for Laetrile." But a study by the American Medical Association's chemical laboratory, compiled two months before the date of the prior paper, indicated success in releasing cyanide during tests with Laetrile. This information did not become public for ten years.

In the interim, media "exposés" of Laetrile — based solely on the incomplete, let alone questionable, 1953 California report — were made. But even a cursory perusal of the 1953 report left much room for doubt. For example, it included an interesting sentence reading: "Thus, all of the physicians whose patients were reviewed spoke of increase in the sense of well-being and appetite, gain in weight and decrease in pain, as though these observations constituted evidence of definitive therapeutic effect."[4] While this statement is susceptible of several interpretations, surely one of them is that the physicians interviewed (apparently by the report writers, the late Doctors Ian MacDonald and Henry L. Garland, chairman and secretary, respectively, of the Cancer Advisory Council) spoke in favor of Laetrile — that is, all of them did, at least up to a point.

Attorney George Kell, defending Albany physician John Richardson on the "cancer quackery" charges, and also defending nutritionist Harvey E. Howard, convicted of practicing medicine without a license by dispensing Laetrile, relied to some extent on the arguments that just such evidences of well-being constitute the very evidence on which physicians rely in order to judge whether, for example, orthodox chemotherapy is a worthwhile palliation.

The 1953 report, the keystone for all subsequent decisions and official opinions on Laetrile, had an ironic follow-up. Doctors MacDonald and Garland (also known for their research report on cigarettes that attempted to invalidate the U.S. surgeon general's report charging cigarette smoking with causing cancer), died in presumptively smoking-connected ways: MacDonald in a fire caused by a lighted cigarette, Garland of cancer of the lung.[5]

As a consequence of the 1953 report, the Laetrile program in the U.S. began to decline. Patients who said they had received help from the substance were not believed. And for most doctors the matter had been solved: Laetrile was one more quack cancer cure, at least in the United States. But abroad, things were different: Dr. Manuel D. Navarro, professor of biochemistry and therapeutics at the University of Santo Tomas, Manila, Philippines, proclaimed Laetrile "the ideal drug for the treatment of cancer." And Dr. Ettore Guidetti of the University of Turin, Italy, reported on the benefits of the direct application of Laetrile to cancer growths, *without having to perform surgery on patients*. His report was a major disclosure at the International Union Against Cancer in 1954.

It was Dr. Navarro who refined an important weapon in cancer detection: the Beard Anthrone Test (BAT), developed by Dr. Howard H. Beard but denied the official blessing of American medical orthodoxy. BAT is said to measure the amount of human chorionic gonadotropin hormone (HCG), appearing in both cancer and pregnancy, in the urine. It had been known that HCG is broken up by the pancreatic enzyme chymotrypsin, and that it rises steadily in the urine of pregnant women until the fifty-sixth day, when it begins to decline; but it rises steadily in the urine of cancer patients until death.

All these were essential points supporting the trophoblastic theory of cancer, the effect of enzymes on cancer, and the efficacy of Laetrile. Dr. Navarro refined to a claimed ninety-seven percent accuracy Dr. Beard's test, and BAT, by positive and negative readings, has become the primary measuring rod for Laetrile cancer therapy.

Despite the curtailing of Laetrile research in the United States, information continued to come in from abroad — England, Belgium, and Japan joining Italy and the Philippines as countries where professional, credentialed researchers were confirming the effectiveness of the substance. Soon, Canada became the focal point of interest in Laetrile, due directly to the intervention of the McNaughton Foundation, then based in Montreal.

Andrew R. L. McNaughton and his foundation (discussed more fully in a later chapter) set up a network of Canadian scientists in liaison with the Canadian government for the official testing of Laetrile, with one savant after another noting and reporting on the effects of the compound. A particular champion was Dr. N. R. Bouziane, professor of pathology and biochemistry at the University of Montreal, dean of the American College of Bioanalysts, and director of research laboratories and chemotherapy specialist of Saint Jeanne D'Arc Hospital's tumor board in Montreal.

Testing and research went on quietly for two years, beginning in 1960. Enthusiasm rippled over Canadian medicine and it seemed that, at last, the answer to cancer had been found.

An American, Dr. John A. Morrone, attending surgeon at the Jersey City Medical Center, on the basis of research in Canada and meetings with Bouziane and Krebs, wrote the first article on Laetrile patients in an American medical journal in 1962, the same year Ernst Krebs, Jr. prepared a lengthy report on his work for both the Canadian and the American food and drug administrations. In *Experimental Medicine and Surgery* (no. 4, 1962), Dr. Morrone, reporting on ten cases, noted a "dramatic relief of pain" in all ten patients after the first or second intravenous injection of Laetrile, with pain vanishing completely in five of the cases. In his summary, he noted pain relief, reduction of the obnoxious odor associated with cancer, improved appetite and reduction of swollen glands, all of which "suggest regression of the malignant lesion."

In the meantime, Judge W. T. Sweigert of the San Francisco Federal District Court allowed limited distribution of supplies of amygdalin (Laetrile) to the McNaughton Foundation in Canada and to several American physicians for investigation with or treatment of patients.

Whether Krebs would get anywhere with the American and Canadian FDAs in legalizing Laetrile for human use essentially turned on an amendment to the original U.S. Food, Drug and Cosmetic Act of 1938 — the "Drug Amendment of 1962," known as the Kefauver Amendment. The amendment was an outgrowth of the worldwide furor over the crippling drug thalidomide, whose sudden mass usage by pregnant women had left a trail of deformed babies.

The amendment added the further requirement of demonstration of drug efficacy in addition to drug safety, a point which overwhelmingly complicated the entire licensing procedure for new drugs and greatly added to what pharmacists and physicians increasingly called the "drug lag" between the United States and the rest of the world.

In order to meet standards for both safety *and* efficacy, a new substance is required to go through a battery of animal studies before it can even be "cleared" for use on human beings. Even then, the FDA guidelines become capricious: If a substance carries with it undoubted possibilities of toxic side effects but is presumed to be effective, and if the effectiveness is thought to overcompensate for the toxicity, then it may literally be rushed on the market — hence the suspicious "legal clearance" of the orthodox cancer chemotherapeutic agents, each one of which *is* a poison, and some of which have been shown actually to *produce* cancer in laboratory animals!

There is some speculation that neither aspirin nor penicillin would be able fully to meet such requirements if required to do so today — inasmuch as penicillin carries with it decidedly dangerous side effects for that part of the population allergic to it; and aspirin has been implicated in the deaths of infants. Laetrile, in the meantime, has never been implicated in anybody's death, has no known toxic side effect, is not a poison, does not cause cancer in laboratory animals, and has now been demonstrated to be of at least some effectiveness in the "treatment, alleviation or prevention" of cancer.

Before returning to the history of Laetrile's suppression we should look at the problem of bureaucracy, particularly following the 1962 amendment to the Food, Drug and Cosmetic Act, since the enormous proliferation of red tape since the passage of this amendment constitutes one of the explanations of Laetrile suppression — regardless of a possible direct conspiracy against the substance. For red tape and bureaucracy are strongly implicated in this nation's "drug lag."

In the October 1973 *Reader's Digest*, an article[6] unearthed these enlightening statistics:

• Since 1963, not a single new general-purpose medicine has been introduced into the U.S. to treat hypertension, even though 23 million Americans are affected by the disease, while between 1967 and 1971 alone five such drugs came into general European practice.

• In the same period, ten medications to treat irregular heartbeat came into the market in Europe, yet by mid-1973 only one of these had been approved for use in the United States.

• At least seven new medications for asthma were introduced in Europe in 1962. By mid-1973 only two could be prescribed in the U.S.A.

• A study conducted by the University of Rochester's Dr. William Wardell found that of the 83 new medicines adopted in both Britain and the U.S. between 1962 and 1971, more than half were introduced in Britain — and an average of 2.8 years elapsed before the FDA allowed them to be sold in this country. During the same time Britain approved for prescription some 80 medications that cannot be prescribed in America, including several that British physicians rate superior to anything available in this country.

The huge jump in paperwork needed to meet pre-and post-1962 FDA requirements is reflected by the fact Parke & Davis, a well-known pharmaceutical company, had to submit 73 pages of evidence to secure the licensing of a drug in 1948, but 20 years later (1968) this had jumped to 72,200 pages of data, transported by truck, simply to license an anesthetic.

Before 1962 it took about six months for a new drug application to be processed, but a decade later this had increased to over 27 months! As a result, the "new chemical entities" (to use the bureaucrats' phrase) coming onto the market fell from 41.5 per year before 1962 to 16.1 in 1970. In 1957-61 some 261 "new drug entities" were produced in the United States, but from 1962 to 1971, twice the amount of time, the total was only 167. In 1961 the U.S. was the world leader in producing new drugs, with 31 (as compared to 9 in France) that year. Over the next eight years, the U.S. introduced only 35 new drugs, while France produced 156.[7]

While this was going on, needed substances were arbitrarily banned in the U.S. DMSO (dimethyl sulfoxide), an effective painkiller developed in the U.S. and used around the world, was arbitrarily banned from use in this country. And, as metabolic physicians advanced the positive use of disodium edetate (EDTA)[8] as a treatment of choice in arteriosclerosis, they found themselves dealing with an "unproven remedy" which, although of orthodox use for treatment in lead poisoning, was now murkily "illegal" because patents on it had expired and compliance for its development under the new FDA guidelines would have cost its promoters millions of dollars.

By 1976, it was generally conceded that to meet the compliance of the FDA "safety" and "efficacy" guidelines in securing the licensing of new "entities," no less than 10 years of trials, both animal and human, nor less than $14 to $15 million in expenditures, nor less than 80,000 pages of paperwork were needed![9]

That is to say, should a company, large or small, or a group of promoters, large or small, attempt to "clear" a new substance through existing bureaucratic machinery, they need an enormous outlay of expenses and a waiting period of up to 10 years before they reach home base. This is an incredible and, to many would-be producers, an impossible situation.

On top of this, what company intends to shell out $15 million for "drug trials" if — as is the case with Laetrile — the product is actually in the public domain and any long-term profit from it is most unlikely?

At the same time, the need for incessant animal studies has been called into question. Dr. Louis Lasagna was quoted in the *Reader's Digest* article already referred to as saying, "you need only a small amount of good clinical work to establish that a drug is effective and reasonably safe. It seems wasteful to spend years getting more data just so people can have a spurious sense of confidence."

And when it wants to be, the FDA can be very "down" on animal tests. When in 1976 a group pressured the agency to ban Flagyl, a drug commonly prescribed for women, on the basis that the substance causes cancer in mice and probably causes cancer in rats as well, the FDA commissioner said: "It is not possible . . . to apply the results of such animal testing directly to humans."

So when the establishment challenged the Laetrile adherents to "secure a license," what was implied was that a substance of already proven benefit, and available limited quantity in two dozen other countries, and already being used by thousands of people, and already backed by several animal studies as well as thousands of testimonials, should start from scratch — and await ten years of trials while an estimated 370,000 people would die *every year* in this country while such tests continued. As we shall see later, Laetrile adherents did make one stab at just such licensing, only to receive a most peculiar response.

The nub of the Laetrilists' legal arguments in the 1970s is that Laetrile, as amygdalin, is not a drug, but a food — specifically, a vitamin — and should not fall under the purview of the FDA's regulatory (rather than legal) ban in the first place, for the only federal provisions against Laetrile, again, do *not* involve a specific law, but an FDA regulation which alerts federal agents to construe Laetrile as either an "unlicensed new drug" or an "unsafe food additive."

The term "drug" is over-broad as it appears in the Food, Drug and Cosmetic Act, which defines any article "intended for use in the diagnosis, cure, mitigation, treatment or prevention of disease" as a "drug." This could, of course, mean that feeding a man suffering from starvation a hamburger could be construed as giving a diseased patient a drug, just as water administered to an individual dying of thirst could also be called a "drug," since it is certainly being used in either the treatment or mitigation of disease.

The belief of Laetrile adherents that they were using a metabolic agent, a specific food with a wide range of effects on the metabolism, rather than a specific substance for a specific treatment, underlies the legal arguments of the 1970s that Laetrile (as Vitamin B-17) constitutes a central substance in nutritional or metabolic therapy, rather than a drug to treat cancer — hence their view that Laetrile should not be within the purview of the FDA to begin with. Even ceding the semantical argument on the over-broad definition of "drug," a chemical (amygdalin) already classified as such and even used therapeutically for well over a century, could hardly be described as a "new drug."

The full vitamin theory of the nitrilosides was not elaborated until 1970, though Krebs' earlier writings suggest he was leaning toward that definition some years before. So Laetrile was still classed in the public mind as a "drug" by March 1963, when the FDA concluded that it "has seen no competent, scientific evidence that Laetrile is effective for the treatment of cancer."

Earlier, Ernst Krebs, Jr. and the John Beard Memorial Foundation he had established in San Francisco pled guilty in U.S. District Court to five counts of violating the "new-drug" provisions of the Food, Drug and Cosmetic Act. A fine of $3,755 was assessed. Imprisonment for Krebs, Jr. was suspended and he was placed on three years' probation, with the provision that he was prohibited from the interstate shipment of all new drugs, including Laetrile, without a new-drug application from the FDA.

Also in 1963 the California State Public Health Department issued a report that essentially upheld the California Cancer Commission's 1953 study, and recommended that the use of Laetrile in cancer therapy be prohibited under the provisions of the 1959 state law that created the Cancer Advisory Council. The report concluded that " 'Laetriles' are of no value in the diagnosis, treatment, alleviation or cure of cancer."

The report further recommended that a regulation be issued prohibiting the use of "Laetriles" (that is, the beta-cyanogenetic glucosides called amygdalin and prunasin) or "substantially similar" agents for such purposes. The regulation was issued September 20, 1963, and became effective November 1, 1963.

With the FDA banning the interstate shipment of Laetrile and the California regulation banning the use of Laetrile in cancer therapy, the home state of Laetrile thus became the state where it was most vigorously opposed.

The McNaughton Foundation apprised the American Cancer Society in 1969 that information had been filed with food and drug officials in the United States, Canada, and Mexico in sufficient quantity "normally . . . adequate for the release of a new drug for clinical testing in humans." It noted that in Mexico an independent preliminary evaluation of Laetrile patients had been carried out "under government auspices with most encouraging results." Indeed, Mexico was soon to become the new focus of Laetrile activity because of the vague legal situation surrounding the compound in the United States.

Amygdalin in its various forms was enjoined from interstate commerce in the United States, when prepared as pharmaceuticals for human medical use. Yet it could be transported interstate when animal testing was the objective. Meanwhile, American doctors were forbidden to hint that Laetrile could be of any value in the treatment or control of cancer.

On August 2, 1965, Ernst Krebs, Sr. agreed to a permanent court injunction against further distribution of the drug, and told the U.S. District Court in San Francisco that he was going out of business. According to the *FDA Report on Enforcement and Compliance*, September 1965, he also "pleaded 'no contest' to criminal contempt charges stating that he disobeyed a restraining order prohibiting shipment of Laetrile in interstate commerce.

"Since the restraining order was issued in May 1965, Dr. Krebs had shipped Laetrile to a hospital in Alabama and to doctors in Utah, Texas, and Washington."

The same report noted that the Canadian Food and Drug Directorate had taken action against the McNaughton Foundation in Canada, contending that the product it was sponsoring "was dangerous and did not meet the requirements of the New-Drug Act, which, similar to U.S. law, requires proof of safety and efficacy."

On January 21, 1966, Dr. Krebs, Sr. pleaded guilty to a contempt charge of shipping Laetrile in violation of an injunction, and on February 3 he was given a one-year suspended sentence by the California U.S. District Court for failing to register as a producer of drugs — particularly Laetrile — coming under the "drug" definition of the Food, Drug and Cosmetics Act.

The legal situation in the United States and Canada, which led the McNaughton Foundation to switch many of its activities to Mexico, by no means halted worldwide interest in the uses of Laetrile. At the quadrennial conference of the International Cancer Congress meeting in Tokyo, Japan, in 1966, the West German M.D., Hans Nieper, first learned about the Krebs compound. Dr. Nieper began administering Laetrile in far greater doses than had been used by Dr. Krebs.

Americans began going to West Germany in the late 1960s to visit Dr. Nieper and to be treated there. These included several very wealthy Americans, some of them wishing to remain anonymous. I personally learned of two of the Nieper cases, one including a rapid reduction in a huge prostatic tumor of a man in his seventies. It was Dr. Nieper who treated comedian Red Buttons' wife before her dramatic announcement in 1973 that her once-terminal cancer was now "controlled" by Laetrile.

But the primary focus of attention for American cancer patients who sought Laetrile turned out to be Tijuana — a name, unfortunately, also associated with quickie divorces and cash-and-carry abortions. Dr. Ernesto Contreras, a graduate of the Mexican Army Medical School who did postgraduate work in Boston, told me in an interview in his new clinic-hospital in Playas de Tijuana that he had learned about Laetrile "by accident" in the early 1960s when Mexican cancer patients had mentioned it to him.

I had interviewed two of Dr. Contreras' patients earlier — both former terminal cases and now Laetrile true-believers — and I expected to find in the gentle Mexican physician an outspoken Laetrile advocate. Instead, all Dr. Contreras was really prepared to say (in interviews ranging from 1972 to 1974) was that Laetrile seemed to be the best of the medical agents available and that by no means was he buying the unitarian trophoblastic theory entirely, even though "that theory holds for ninety percent of the cases of cancer."

The clinic, which is daily filled with patients, most of them Americans, was operating on legal, if just barely legal, status in 1972, before Laetrile had secured the full official blessing of the Mexican government. That blessing it obtained in 1973. Californians spoke of the "Laetrile underground," whereby patients from throughout the country made the trip to Tijuana, usually via San Diego, or were otherwise able to procure Laetrile from Mexico.

Most of the Laetrile consumed in the United States was coming from a Tijuana laboratory. Costs of the substance were modest compared with prices for U.S. cancer drugs, and treatment and hospitalization in Tijuana were modest, too, even though the virtual monopoly of American terminal cancer patient traffic in Tijuana left many people with an assembly-line impression of the operation there. As of 1974, Dr. Contreras told me, about a thousand new patients per year, or between 100 and 120 patients per month, were visiting his Del Mar Clinic — a figure which was ballooning by 1976.[10] The Mexican medic had a large staff, including ten other doctors and expanding facilities. As of 1976, the Del Mar Clinic was the largest of four clinics in Tijuana in which Laetrile therapy was available, and its caseload was mushrooming to 5,000 a year.

As of 1972, Dr. Contreras said he had personally treated 2,500 cancer patients in Tijuana with Laetrile. That figure had doubled by 1976, and was only a portion of the thousands of patients who had visited the increasingly famous clinic since 1963. The American Medical Association and California food and drug officials estimated the total as high as 55,000 persons.[11]

In interviews with me, however, Dr. Contreras at all times chose his words carefully. He admitted his clinic was established to treat patients, not keep records; that records of some patients were more complete than others; that followup of many patients was difficult. His "Preliminary Report" of 500 cases between 1963 and 1967 indicated "beneficial effects" in 64 percent of cases against 36 percent showing no such response.[12] By 1976, Dr. Contreras was claiming a 67% "positive response" in 5,000 cases, based on 10,000 sets of medical records of his patients over a fourteen-year period.

Dr. Contreras at no time claimed he was offering a "cure" for cancer — at best his approach offered a "control," he told me. Although Dr. Contreras mixed both orthodox and "unorthodox" therapies in treating cancer, by 1976 he was increasingly using the total metabolic approach (other vitamins, enzymes, a special diet) as suggested for Laetrile patients.

The "responses" he saw in patients after 14 years of using Laetrile ranged from the increase in well-being and general cessation of cancer-connected pain — the most consistent Laetrile response reported to me over several years by several score patients — and the regaining of normal color, appetite and weight, to actual remissions of all symptoms.

Few of his patients had undergone what Dr. Contreras termed "total control" of their cancers. Thirty-five percent had experienced no response at all, and of the sixty-five percent who did evince some benefit from Laetrile, almost half had had recurrences of the disease after its temporary arrest. For this group, inability to arrest tumors or provoke their remission was typical, he said. For the remaining thirty percent, in the "more definite responses" category, results ranged from slight improvement to the dramatic disappearance of all symptoms. A patient is considered "controlled" after five symptom-free years but remains on pill maintenance dosages for the rest of his or her life, much as a diabetic must remain on insulin.

The salient characteristic about the Contreras therapy then (and the Richardson treatments later) is that up to ninety percent of his cases, almost all of them Americans, are terminal cancer patients — persons given weeks, months, a year at most to survive. The Mexican physician repeated the Krebs view that Laetrile is no miracle cure, that it cannot restore damaged tissues. All it can do, and even then not in all cases, is to attack and destroy cancer cells while building up the body's natural defenses against the disease. Noting that his therapy "may have saved five percent of the terminal cases I have seen," Dr. Contreras added that for the great number of other patients, months and even years had been added to their lives even though death eventually overtook them.

The Contreras clinic and hospital were in the news frequently from 1970 on; the alternate successes and failures of patients headed for "the

Tijuana connection" were monitored whenever possible. Most Contreras patients, following massive intravenous Laetrile injections, are sent home with Laetrile tablets and orders for a strict diet, since laetrilists regard the need for a select diet as important as Laetrile itself. A slippage in diet was accompanied by a return of tumors in numerous cases I learned about.

The Mexican doctor said there is no proof yet that Laetrile is a cancer preventative, but added that it "most probably" is. He soft-pedaled the preventative use of Laetrile, arguing that there was not yet enough of it available even for all the cancer-sick patients.

He exhibited bitterness and frustration over what he called "the FDA campaign against Laetrile." He asserted that "it meets all the requirements asked by the FDA [for clearance for human use] — they have all been filled by Laetrile." Federal officials continued to deny this, and even alleged that Dr. Contreras and his staff did not comply with requests to make available thorough, solid Laetrile case histories.

While Contreras' treatment continued to be known by word of mouth and intermittent press reports, the McNaughton Foundation continued to fight for permission to test Laetrile; its dossier was jammed with cases from many foreign sources, including the Contreras ones. The strange switch of 1970 then occurred.

In April 1970 the Food and Drug Administration assigned IND (Investigative New Drug) application number 6734 to the McNaughton Foundation, based in California, to test amygdalin-Laetrile, a move which would have given the foundation permission to obtain supplies of the "investigational drug" and to initiate clinical studies. Then, ten days later, permission was suddenly revoked by the FDA, allegedly at the behest of the then surgeon general Jesse Steinfeld, a California physician involved in the California Medical Association ban on the compound in the 1950s.[13] Dr. Charles C. Edwards, FDA commissioner, stated on June 9, 1970:

> *As with all "cancer" drugs the review of the IND was expedited. . . . This review was completed on April 27, 1970, 21 days from the date of receipt. The review disclosed a number of serious preclinical deficiencies.*
>
> *On April 28, 1970, a 10-day pretermination notice was issued detailing the deficiencies in the notice, and the sponsor was notified by wire to immediately cease clinical studies. The sponsor was allowed 10 days in which to either request a conference or to correct the deficiencies which were brought to his attention.*
>
> *Since the sponsor did neither, the IND was terminated on May 12, 1970.[14]*

This is the kind of statement tailored to enrage Dr. Dean Burk,

Laetrile's single key friend inside the government structure. The head of the National Cancer Institute's cytochemistry division said in a May 30, 1972, letter to Rep. Louis Frey: "I may add that I have been reliably informed by the staff member in charge of handling IND applications in one of the largest cancer research organizations in the country that the Mc-Naughton Foundation IND application 6734 is superior in content and extent to most all of the IND applications made by and granted to said research organization, and this in spite of the report of the 'kangaroo court and jury' of the FDA."

Also, although the McNaughton Foundation was given only ten days to remedy the "deficiencies," and although its new supporting data were in the mail within that deadline, the FDA claimed the Foundation had failed to comply; its IND denial remained in effect.

Dr. Burk, a thirty-four-year veteran of government service in his field, was the primary heavyweight to come over to the Laetrile camp, not because he thought Laetrile was the final answer or because of any devotion to the trophoblastic theory, but because he found his own testing of it on mice to be effective and "absolutely nontoxic." He battled for years against an orthodox medical and pharmaceutical establishment that promoted "official" but highly toxic anticancer drugs with low levels of success in therapy while consistently thwarting clinical testing on humans of Laetrile and other allegedly nontoxic anticancer substances.

Backers, supporters, and users of Laetrile were once again puzzled, as were, finally, some of the U.S. media. If Laetrile was worthless, why not openly, officially, clinically test it on humans and find out? Were the reports of medical men like Contreras, Nieper, Bouziane, and Navarro really without foundation? Were thousands of users deluded into believing they were having some relief with the apricot-kernel extract? Yet, only silence greeted such questions, and more and more sustained Ernst Krebs, Jr.'s longheld thesis that the "chief harassment" against Laetrile emanated from state food and drug agencies at the behest of the FDA.

On September 1, 1971, the FDA said in a news release that an Ad Hoc Committee on Consultants for Review and Evaluation of Laetrile had found "no acceptable evidence of therapeutic effect to justify clinical trials" of the drug. The blue-ribbon panel[15] findings preceded the news release, which stated:

> *Under the FDA position reinforced today by the Ad Hoc Committee findings, Laetrile (amygdalin) may not be promoted, tested or sold in the United States under provisions of the Federal Food, Drug and Cosmetic Act until the necessary basic studies have been accomplished. The FDA also has requested Dr. Ernesto Contreras, Mexico, and*

Dr. Hans Nieper, Germany, to provide any clinical records they may have on Laetrile treatments they have been giving patients.

The FDA said the request was part of its continuing efforts to obtain scientific evidence to support claims by Laetrile advocates that the substance is an effective anticancer agent.

So the clampdown was official as far as the FDA was concerned. Empowered to rule on "new drugs," semantically equipped to regard a food used in the treatment of a disease as a "drug," and able to control interstate shipments, the FDA tightened the noose around Laetrile.

This was the background to the Richardson arrest and the mass proliferation of committees sprouting up nationwide. They repeatedly asked the key question: Why *not* test Laetrile? One government-baiting attorney, Washington's John Joseph Matonis, aiding several of the legal cases on several fronts, believed:

The FDA's legal authority — if indeed it is legal — is unconstitutionally applied in the case of Laetrile and nutritional remedies for cancer. The FDA is unfairly discriminating against Laetrile by enforcing standards higher than those established for other drugs which are more in alignment with FDA's philosophy.

They say Laetrile is banned because it's not effective — which it certainly is — but then they allow a variety of other drugs that are extremely poisonous, and not necessarily effective.[16]

Despite the clampdown, Laetrile use continued growing at a geometric rate, spurred not only by the rapid growth of the Committee for Freedom of Choice in Cancer Therapy, Inc., which grew in four years from a single chapter and five members to more than 400 chapters and 28,000 members, but because of the worsening cancer statistics and virtual admission, if *sub rosa*, by clinicians that "orthodox" cancer cures were failing.

Thousands more patients streamed to Tijuana, where the CytoPharma de Mexico laboratory produced most of the high-grade Laetrile being used in North America. By 1976 the general estimate was that between 35,000 and 50,000 Americans and Canadians were either "on" or had been using Laetrile.

In Tijuana, not only had Dr. Contreras' facilities, staff and practice greatly expanded, but the Del Rio brothers, operators of CytoPharma (originally established with the collaboration of Andrew McNaughton), had opened Clinica Cydel, whose medical director, Dr. Mario Soto de Leon, had already helped pioneer the use of Laetrile in Mexico City at the 20 de Noviembre Hospital.

Starting out with careful attention to statistics, records-keeping and guidelines acceptable to the Mexican version of the FDA, Cydel claimed by spring 1976 that a cluster of cases selected for thoroughness of stateside diagnosis, treatment in Mexico, confirmation both inside and outside the U.S., and adequate followup, showed overwhelming response to Laetrile therapy.

The author was allowed to see most of the records of these 100 cases (of some 180 patients treated at Cydel since fall 1975) and saw evidence of complete control of cancer crises through the use of Laetrile (B-17) as the *single* cancer-fighting agent involved; control of a brain tumor through daily 12-gram Laetrile doses; dramatic remission of adenocarcinoma in a woman given one to two months to live in 1975 before visiting Cydel; the stopping of the spread of a melanoma with 12-gram Laetrile injections; a variety of positive responses while mixing large doses of Laetrile with smaller injections of toxic chemotherapies in 20 cases, including three dramatic regressions of lymphoma.[17]

Dr. Soto was able to reconfirm his own clinical evidence in several cases by having them "scanned" by the Nuclear Medicine Department of the University of California-San Diego Hospital — a practice which was mysteriously curtailed by the stateside facility as of spring 1976.

In the United States, of some 800 physician-members of the Committee for Freedom of Choice in Cancer Therapy, Inc., by 1976 between 40 and 50 were openly using Laetrile in their practices — far from the half-dozen or so medics who were using the substance, usually in secret, four years earlier.

Dr. E. Paul Wedel of Oregon, himself a recovered Laetrile cancer patient and an outstanding metabolic physician, reported positive benefits from Vitamin B-17 as a key part of nutritional or metabolic therapy in almost 4,000 cases. Such physicians as Philip Binzel of Ohio, Raymond Hillyard of North Carolina, and S. R. "Pete" Abramson of Louisiana were openly using Laetrile as nutritional therapy and reporting excellent results. Embattled California pioneer John A. Richardson, a victor in three State of California trials and the subject of continual harassment by federal and state officials, continued using Laetrile in his metabolic practice, with some 6,000 cases treated by 1976.

Only in California did Laetrile remain specifically illegal for use in cancer therapy, but pressure from above was applied in several other states through the threat of "peer review" — *i.e.*, enforced appearances of physicians before their state medical boards and the risk of their licenses for daring to use "unproven cancer remedies" in their practices. In Alabama, for example, a gifted physician who had rescued many Southerners from death's door through the Laetrile program, was undergoing the possible loss of his license from the state medical board if he did not cease and desist in the use of Laetrile.

In other parts of the world, Dr. Hans Nieper of West Germany continued reporting favorable success with Laetrile in the form of "activated amygdalin" and Drs. Goenawan and Simandjuntak from Indonesia reported on the successful use of San Pedro Petro cassava (bitter cassava), a plant bearing considerable Vitamin B-17, on some 6,000 cancer patients — paralleling the work of Asian Laetrile pioneer Dr. Manuel Navarro of Manila, who was finding Vitamin B-17 efficacy not only from the product Laetrile but as a prevention in the form of the natural substance cassava, which is a staple food in the Philippines.

Evidence that the therapeutic product Laetrile (in vial and tablet form, and as the natural Vitamin B-17 found in a wide variety of plants, seeds and vegetables) constitutes not only a *preferred* treatment of cancer and other conditions, but may very well be the *primary* preventative of cancer, was gathering monthly.

CHAPTER EIGHT

The Cyanide Hunters

SINCE THE ALLEGED ACTION of cyanide is the presumptive retardant of cancer in Laetrile, and because free cyanide is indeed poison, American public health authorities have been able to frighten the public about Laetrile simply by using the word "cyanide" often enough. The fear of cyanide also underlies the official attacks — some seemingly with a touch of tongue in cheek — against apricot kernels themselves and two nitriloside-bearing products called "Aprikern" and "Bee Seventeen."

Dr. Krebs and other researchers have noted the presence of cyanide in one form or another in many of the foods we eat. More important, it occurs very much in the early evolutionary process. Laetrilists were cheered to note that astronomers examining the passage of the comet Kohoutek in December-January 1973-74 detected as an "unusual" feature of the massive heavenly body the presence of hydrogen cyanide, cosmic proof of the considerable cyanide presence in the formative processes of solar systems.

I wondered, at the time,. if the presence of Kohoutek and the detection of hydrogen cyanide in the gigantic celestial wanderer were not somehow symbolic of the battles being fought on Earth over Laetrile, for its visible presence paralleled the months of extreme agitation on the legal, scientific, and propaganda fronts of the onrushing Laetrile battle.

While Laetrile was banned for sale at the FDA level not on the basis of toxicity but on the allegation that it simply is worthless as a cancer treatment, lower-level attacks by officialdom, usually thinly veiled, insinuated the danger of cyanide. ("Tests show that Laetrile is forty times as toxic when taken by mouth as when given by injection," noted the former executive secretary of the California Advisory Council in officially sanctioned material on cancer quackery.) No matter that the National Cancer Institute's Dr. Dean Burk routinely denounced these fears as baseless, styling the apricot kernel extract "less toxic than sugar." No matter that Krebs, as part of his voluminous research on the nitrilosides and toxicity, found huge presumptive levels of tolerance for the poison — usually safe in nature's compounds — in animals. And no matter that not a single authenticated case of cyanosis fatality was known in the quarter century that Laetrile, in one form or another, has been used in humans.

The whole matter of cyanide in apricot kernels or in other seeds or in Laetrile has been one of the major red herrings in the Laetrile story. McNaughton Foundation president Andrew McNaughton noted[1] that "after all, amygdalin has been around for at least 3,000 years — the ancient Chinese used bitter almonds, with properties similar to those in the apricot seed, as a medicine. But bitter almonds, by agreement with the U.S. Food and Drug Administration, are not on the American market because one of the elements is cyanide — and FDA thinks cyanide will kill you."

Which of course it can — if it's in free form and a necessary amount. But according to McNaughton, the developers of Laetrile, and the researchers on amygdalin around the world, cyanide naturally occurring in food is not dangerous. Primitive peoples who eat only natural, organic and "unfractionated" foods, they claim, daily take in anywhere from 250 to 500 milligrams of organic cyanide. But the natural cyanide — as is claimed to be the chemical case for Laetrile or any version of amygdalin — is locked in a sugar molecule. This natural cyanide, they say, is normal to human metabolism, and is found in over 1,200 unrefined foods and grasses. When eaten, an enzyme (rhodanese) is said to detoxify the cyanide and it is eliminated through the body's normal processes.

The California pressure against the dispensing of apricot kernels in health-food stores — and apricot kernels were routinely sold in such stores as the Golden State led the nation in the health-food mania — paralleled the arrest of Dr. Richardson and his first trial. For a time, some health-food store operators simply removed their packages of the kernels, the almondlike nuts broken out of the tough apricot pit, from front-room view to the backroom. But by 1976 it became difficult to find such packages; obviously the gradual spread of fear was producing results.

In September 1972 the California State Department of Public Health issued a warning that the eating of apricot kernels could cause cyanide poisoning and even death. This came as health-food stores were selling the dry kernels for $1 per pound and up.

I caught up with this particular ramification of the overall story on Monday, September 5, after a wire service had carried the "warning." It was based on the experience of an unnamed Los Angeles couple who had reportedly gotten sick from eating a concoction of apricot seeds mixed with dried apricots and distilled water, put through a blender, and left overnight. The reported illness preceded the health department statement and provided the immediate effect of bringing into question the cyanide content of apricot kernels and of many other seeds. While Laetrile was not mentioned, the inference to be drawn seemed plain — for, again, the specific chemical action on cancer tumors claimed by Laetrile boosters is the release by a specific enzyme of the cyanide contained in the cyanide-benzaldehyde-glucose compound that is Laetrile.

I immediately contacted Dr. Ben Werner, the department's epidemiologist, and Dr. Ralph Weilerstein, then the department's public medical officer and an outspoken foe of Laetrile. "Death from this is probably rare and even when it occurs may not be diagnosed as cyanide poisoning from overeating of such kernels," Dr. Werner told me. I wanted to know, since the department was quoted in the media as implying the possibility not only of cyanide poisoning but also of death, if *any* such cases had actually been discovered in California or the rest of the United States. The answer from both men was that no cases of cyanide fatalities from eating apricot kernels were known. Indeed, I was finally told, the suggestion of such fatalities came from a British medical journal referring to a vague case in Turkey, more than a decade earlier, involving symptoms "suggesting" cyanide poisoning. I was also referred to a British report on African tribes that consume large amounts of fruit kernels and are said to suffer the symptoms of cyanide poisoning.

Actually, the only worldwide reports of such poisoning come from two fatalities of presumptive cyanide poisoning out of nine cases reported at the Children's Hospital of the Hacettepe Medical Center, Ankara, in 1957, and four cases of presumptive cyanide poisoning — none fatal — reported during a 22-year span at the Institute of Medico-Legal Research in Bucarest, Rumania. Both these sets of cases were reported in the *New England Journal of Medicine* for May 21, 1964,[2] and hardly make an overwhelming case against the ingestion of apricot, or any other, kernels.

To begin with, the Turkish cases deal exclusively with children, whose ages ranged from 2½ to 5 years. I was told that the two fatalities probably were poor waifs who rummaged through garbage and consumed a good many things, among which *may have been* apricot kernels. The Bucarest studies constitute the only reported instances in Europe that I know of — and the article is careful to state that "reports of actual poisoning from seed sources among humans are not frequent."

Suffice it to say that if there were only 13 cases of possible efficacy in cancer from Laetrile over a 22-year period of experience on one whole continent and part of another, Laetrile adherents would be laughed out of the clinic by asserting positive Laetrile effects from such statistics — yet, we are supposed to recoil in terror when we read of 13 such cases of *presumptive* cyanide poisoning, including two fatalities, from apricot kernels in the 22-year experience of one continent and one other country!

Dr. Werner agreed that "not enough is known" about apricot kernels and those of other fruits, except that "too many" might bring about symptoms of cyanosis. But no one seemed to know how many "too many" are.

I did not then, and do not now, scorn health officials for occasionally issuing unintentionally misleading statements about food. After all, the health-food craze was being revved up with a vengeance in the late 1960s and early 1970s, and was a major part of the "counterculture." That back-to-nature young people might be hurting themselves through consuming uncommon blends of unusual foods was not particularly surprising; after all, this was the era of the demonstrably dangerous "macrobiotic diet" of certain Zen and allied cultists.

The official federal line on Laetrile remained the same: It is not poisonous, only worthless. Nonetheless, stimulus-response words like "cyanide" and "toxicity" kept cropping up in California health department discussions of Laetrile, reaching a point in 1973 in which a state medical journal article left the impression that a Laetrile user was literally taking his life in his hands by turning to the "worthless" substance.

Jay Hutchinson, who, like many Laetrile users and true-believers, is a fearless opponent of medical orthodoxy, provided an anecdote to the California drive against apricot kernels. Aware that the oft-described Hunza people of the "Shangri-la" valleys of the Himalayas are vigorous consumers of apricots in every form, Hutchinson addressed the royal Mir and Rhani of Hunzaland thus in an airmail special-delivery letter:

> I am rushing this extremely urgent warning to you so that you can take immediate steps to notify your government and your people of the health hazard reported by the California State Department of Public Health during the week of September 3, 1972.
>
> I enclose articles from San Francisco newspapers ... it is obvious that this is serious and that no humor was intended (we have heard that you and your wife, the Rhani, have a great sense of humor).
>
> As you can see this is not the time for humor — rather, it is a time for action. Mir, you must get your people to stop eating those pits! Stop making flour out of them! Stop feeding your newborn infants the oil, and for Mohammed's sake, stop anointing them with it!
>
> I feel certain that the California State Department of Public Health (fraud division) would provide you with copious data proving you have been poisoning yourselves these many hundreds of years!
>
> Please write soon, and when you do, would you mind telling us why your people are among the healthiest in the world, and why your men and women live vigorous lives well into their 90s, and why you and your beautiful people never get cancer?

Renee Taylor told of the amazing health, vitality and longevity of the Hunzakuts in her book, *Hunza Health Secrets*. In it she recalls how the

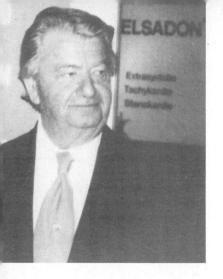

Ernst T. Krebs, Jr., the pioneer co-discoverer of vitamins B-15 and B-17, is one of this century's major innovators in science. A biochemist with several hundred citations in medical literature and several patents in his name for his work in science, Krebs risked the wrath of the medical/pharmaceutical/governmental establishment with the vitamin-deficiency theory of cancer.

Ernst T. Krebs, Sr., M.D., a physician who once made his rounds with a horse and buggy, was a medical innovator whose footsteps would later be followed by his son. A free thinker with a fighting spirit, the late Dr. Krebs first learned of the amazing properties of Laetrile, or vitamin B-17, while searching for a way to make bootleg whiskey taste better.

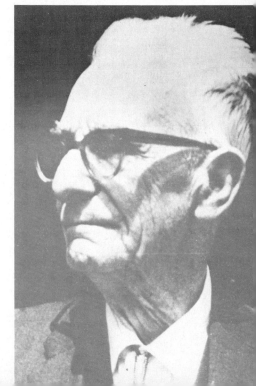

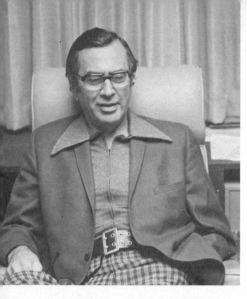

Andrew R. L. McNaughton, the British-born scion of a prominent Canadian family, has been at the center of the Laetrile hurricane for many years. A bold and courageous adventurer, whose varied career has included gun-running for the founders of Israel and later the Castro movement in Cuba, McNaughton organized a foundation to assist innovative medical research. When Laetrile was outlawed in California, and indirectly banned in the rest of the United States, it was the McNaughton Foundation that was responsible for continuing the research and development of this remarkable substance.

Dean Burk, Ph.D. was a founder of the National Cancer Institute and for years was the chief of its cytochemistry division. A researcher with a worldwide reputation, Dr. Burk was a skeptic who became an ardent advocate of Laetrile. Until his retirement in 1974, he was virtually

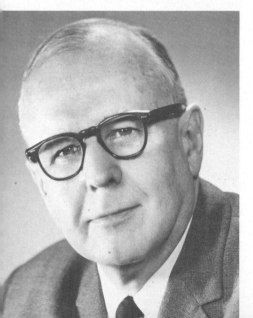

the sole voice within the "establishment" battling for the credibility of vitamin B-17. A witty speaker and trenchant writer, Dr. Burk accused medical and governmental orthodoxy of juggling figures and manipulating statistics in order to support claims that Laetrile was worthless.

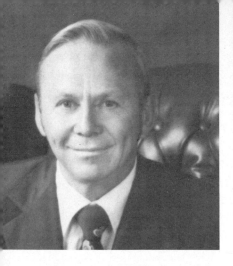
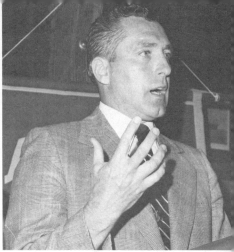

Robert W. Bradford (above, left), an electronics engineer and physicist earlier associated with the Stanford Linear Accelerator, gave up a lucrative career as head of his own electronics firm to become President of the Committee for Freedom of Choice in Cancer Therapy. Under his leadership, the grassroots movement grew in less than four years to over 400 chapters and 28,000 members.

John A. Richardson, M.D. (above, right) was the first American physician to announce publicly that he used Laetrile in his practice — even after the substance was technically outlawed. Arrested and harassed through three court trials, the California physician won acquittal on all charges, enabling his patients to continue receiving vitamin B-17.

Four spokesmen for the Committee for Freedom of Choice in Cancer Therapy (below) address a California press conference to answer some of the vicious allegations against Laetrile and its supporters. From left to right, committee members Dr. Ernst T. Krebs, Jr., Dr. John A. Richardson, Mike Culbert, and Robert W. Bradford respond.

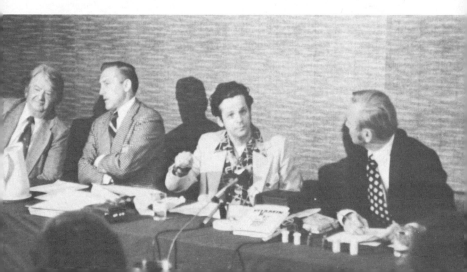

E. Paul Wedel, M.D. (right) is both a "controlled" Laetrile cancer patient and a metabolic physician with an outstanding reputation. By mid-1976, Dr. Wedel had treated over 3,500 cancer victims, almost all of whom had been considered terminal. As a result of his program of total metabolic therapy, more than half of his patients are still alive — a success ratio several times higher than that of "orthodox" medical treatment.

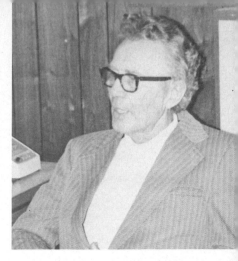

Beverly Newkirk, Executive Director of the Committee for Freedom of Choice in Cancer Therapy, helped put the organization on the map by organizing symposia and doctors' conferences across the country. She also researched many cancer-prevention diets, a number of which appear in this book.

The discoverer of pangamic acid (vitamin B-15), as well as Laetrile, Dr. Ernst T. Krebs, Jr., is shown below before a commercial display in West Germany promoting the substance. But medical reports in this country credit the Soviet Union for the development of pangamic acid.

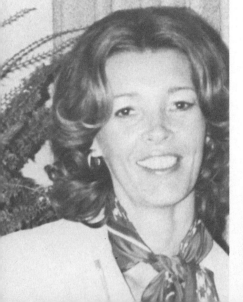

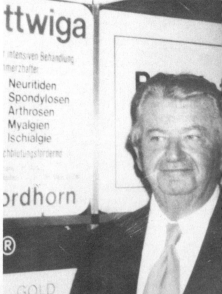

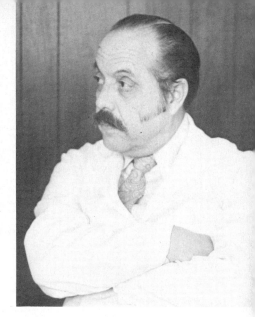

Ernesto Contreras, M.D. is perhaps the best-known Laetrile physician in the world. In the past decade, thousands of American cancer patients flocked to his Del Mar Medical Center in Tijuana, Mexico, for a treatment that was legal in Mexico but condemned in the United States. After fourteen years of experience with Laetrile, by 1976 Dr. Contreras had assembled thousands of case histories of remarkable recoveries.

Manuel D. Navarro, M.D. has worked with Laetrile for over 24 years at the Santo Tomas University Hospital research center in Manila, the Philippines. He is best known for refining the test for cancer by measuring the amount of human chorionic gonadotropin (HCG) in the urine.

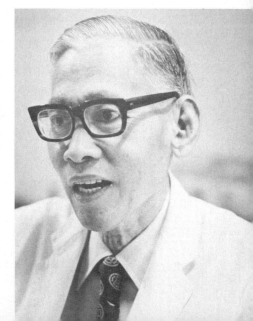

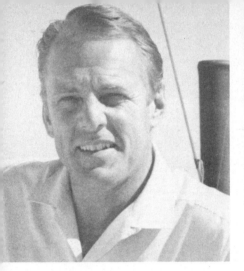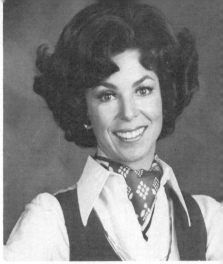

Frank Salaman, founding member and Vice President of the Committee for Freedom of Choice in Cancer Therapy, assisted the Del Rio brothers in establishing the Cydel Clinic for holistic metabolic medicine in 1975. He was one of the key figures in helping the Committee grow to over 28,000 members and 400 chapters across the nation.

Maureen Salaman, co-editor of The Choice, the monthly magazine of the Committee, is active in promoting legislative programs for the legalization of Laetrile. She is noted for her positive and powerful arguments and articles on behalf of freedom of choice.

A major legal breakthrough for Laetrile advocates occurred in December 1975, when "terminal" cancer patient Glen Rutherford (below, center) won the right in a court case in Oklahoma to import Laetrile from Mexico. Congratulating Rutherford on his victory are Committee for Freedom of Choice in Cancer Therapy officers Robert W. Bradford (below, right) and Franklin Salaman (below, left).

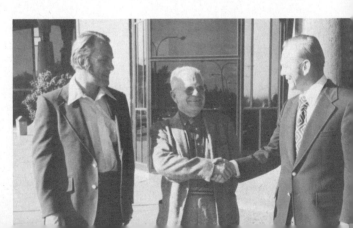

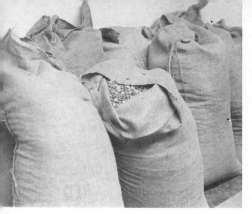

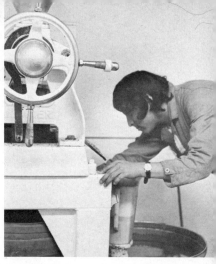

Laetrile in the making is shown in these photographs taken at the CytoPharma de Mexico laboratory. Bags of apricot kernels (above, left) arrive at the warehouse, where they are ground and defatted with a cold solvent (above, right). When the solvent is removed from the ground pulp, the resulting powder is then added to boiling alcohol (below, right), the mix is carefully filtered, and amygdalin is extracted. The filtrate is then frozen and Laetrile crystals are recovered.

Mexican supplies of Laetrile were established when Jorge Del Rio (below, left) opened the Cyto-Pharma de Mexico factory in Tijuana. Later, Del Rio and his brothers started the Cydel Clinic in Tijuana, with oncologist Mario Soto de Leon (below, right) as its medical director.

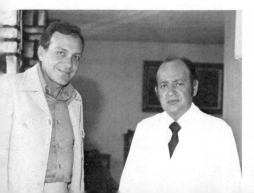

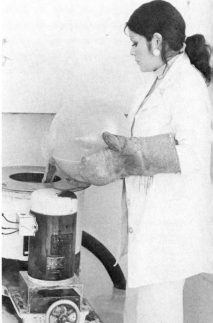

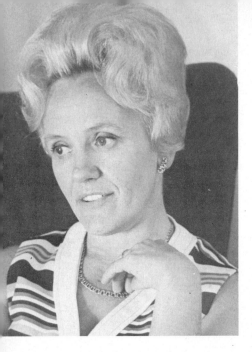

Three benefactors of the Laetrile movement are Mrs. Joan Wilkinson (left), who turned to Laetrile in 1968 after two previous operations failed to "get it all." Told that her left leg and hip should be amputated, by 1969 she was pronounced free of cancer. Mrs. Betty Elder (below, left), who suffered more from "orthodox" chemotherapy treatment than she did from cancer, is now a fervent Laetrile advocate who credits the substance with saving her life. A coed from High Point, North Carolina, Pam McDaniel (below, right) was told in March 1975 that she could not expect to see Christmas that year, because of terminal, metastasized bone cancer. After treatment with Laetrile, Miss McDaniel was free of pain and cancer in 1976.

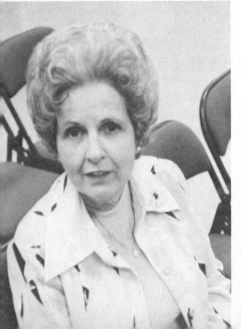

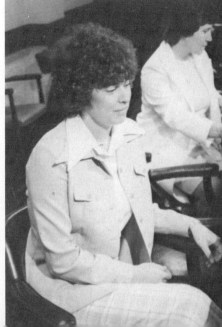

Hunzakut women found a supplementary source of fat in milk-scarce Hunzaland in the seed of the apricot, and how the knowledge of how to use it had passed from mother to daughter down through the centuries.

"Since apricot oil is so essential for their diet, every farmer grows more apricot trees than any of the other fruit trees," she wrote. "It is even said that the maiden's choice of a husband depends on how many apricot trees he owns." She added, "Today the apricot is not only the most popular fruit, it is also the most versatile. Its oil is used in cooking, salad dressings, as a food supplement and for medicine, and it is even used as a cosmetic on their skin and hair. Men, women and children use this oil, and it is obvious that it brings excellent results, as most all of them have beautiful skin and lovely hair."[3]

She describes how apricots are made into paste, jam, bread, and juice, and how it is common for the Hunzakuts to eat apricots, crack open their pits with their teeth (no mean task), and consume the seeds within.

Despite reports that Hunzaland is not really the utopia some dreamers claim it to be and that some cases of Hunza cancer have been noted, Prince Mohammed Ameen Khan, son of the Mir, stated flatly to the *Los Angeles Times* on May 6, 1973, that "cancer is unheard of" in Hunzaland.

Retained by the California state apricot industry as a consultant, the twenty-three-year-old prince said the Hunzakuts, whose average life expectancy is eighty-five, eat fresh apricots three months out of the year and dried apricots the rest of the time, also "relishing the apricot nut inside the kernel." Moreover, the people of this remote, 600-square-mile valley, 8,000 feet above sea level, drink apricot juice and cook with apricot oil.

A problem that Laetrile supporters grappled with for some time was how to get the substance out from under the onus of "drug" classification. Their view is that Laetrile is a vitamin, a food factor, and should be treated as such. So in 1973 two products bearing the substance designated vitamin B-17 were introduced into the California market and spread across the country: "Aprikern," manufactured in capsules, and "Bee Seventeen," a powdery, milkshake-like product. The food distributors did not hide the fact that their products were indeed a form of edible Laetrile.

After months of circulation of the products in various states, during which three million capsules of Aprikern and 100,000 packages of Bee Seventeen were sold, the FDA finally struck. On November 23, 1973, Sam D. Fine, the FDA's associate commissioner for compliance, informed Alex Geczy, president of General Research Laboratories, Van Nuys, California:

> *Sample analysis by the Food and Drug Administration of your Aprikern capsules and "Bee" Seventeen product reveals that each con-*

tains hydrogen cyanide in such quantities that they are dangerous. For example, Aprikern capsules were found to contain an average level of over two (2) milligrams hydrogen cyanide per capsule. At that level, the ingestion of only five (5) capsules could be fatal to a child due to cyanide poisoning. Twenty (20) capsules could be fatal to an adult. Oral toxity studies performed on rats support these figures. Likewise, we estimate that the contents of only two (2) packets of the "Bee" Seventeen product could be fatal if ingested by a small child.

Due to not only the inadequacy of the labeling, but also the inherent danger these products pose both to children and adults, forthright action must be taken.

Therefore, in the interest of consumer protection, it will be necessary to completely recall both the Aprikern capsules and the "Bee" Seventeen product from consumer channels.[4]

The ordering off the shelves of such products got under way in California, New York, New Jersey, and Minnesota. The distributors of the products charged "harassment." General Research Laboratories' attorney Stephen Tornay of San Diego argued that the new FDA move was in reality a veiled new tactic against Laetrile and that the federal agency "has no court order and no scientific findings as a basis on which they make assertions."[5] Moreover, Tornay said he had received ambivalent statements from the FDA about the scientific basis for the clampdown against the two products.

The National Cancer Institute's Dr. Dean Burk jumped into the battle almost immediately. He consulted all concerned, including scientists from the College of Pharmacy, University of Arizona, under whose responsibility the tests of the two products were carried out. In a letter to Geczy, Burk said:

In my opinion, the FDA and FDA-derived press reports that Aprikern capsules contained on the average over 2 milligrams of hydrogen cyanide per capsule are grossly in error, and, as reported by the FDA, are both highly misleading and indeed fraudulent with respect to alleged danger to humans eating the capsules . . . .

In other words, the hydrogen cyanide was measured only after several hours of neutral hydrolysis in a large volume of water, under a set of conditions ordinarily never met with in the swallowing of Aprikern capsules by humans, including the condition of stomach acidity precluding enzymatic hydrolysis of amygdalin by betaglucosidase contained in the Aprikern but promptly destroyed by the stomach acidity.

In point of fact, as I have found in my laboratory, the amount of hydrogen cyanide, as such, in Aprikern capsules is negligible in terms of the amounts alleged by the FDA. Thus, the theoretical calculations of the FDA as to the number of capsules that "could be fatal" to adults or children (allegedly 20 and 5 capsules, respectively), based on alleged contents of hydrogen cyanide in the capsules, are scientifically unwarranted . . . .

If such excellently nutritious food as Aprikern were to be recalled from consumer channels, as Mr. Fine's letter indicates, then to avoid discrimination, this might well be equally true of meat, milk, eggs, gelatin, and a great variety of protein-containing foods, all of which have long been known to produce hydrogen cyanide when acted upon by suitable catalytic or enzymatic agents *(bacterially or fungally derived) just as in the case of Aprikern, but under conditions* . . . not ordinarily involved in human usage and consumption.[6]

Nonetheless, the propaganda damage was done and many healthfood store operators went along with the clear-the-shelves order of the Food and Drug Administration. As of April 1974, Aprikern and Bee Seventeen were no longer available.

Aside from the protestations of Dean Burk and the extensive research done by Ernst Krebs, Jr., substantial modern research has tended to bear out the nontoxicity of amygdalin, the chemical name for Laetrile. German researcher Herbert M. Summa's 1972 study, with forty-two citations of scientific research papers, states: "Amygdalin is not toxic and has no negative side effects. It may therefore be administered over [a] long period of time."[6] Such statements collide directly with those of California public health spokesmen, who have suggested a danger in Laetrile due to presumptive toxicity. Again, however, the primary American arguments lodged against amygdalin therapy in cancer treatment are not that the chemical is toxic — simply that it is worthless.

By 1976, the cyanide hunters were at it again — and why not? The hoked-up toxicity statistics on Aprikern and Bee Seventeen, in which large enormous doses of prehydrolyzed material were administered to rats to kill them, had proven to the Feds that they could hoodwink the public and get away with it. Two more non-fatal "cyanide poisoning" cases from apricot kernels were allegedly unearthed by watchful agents in California in 1975, and the "California morbidity report" on them was dispatched throughout the country.

In one case, an individual was said to have developed symptoms of cyanide poisioning by eating a "handful" of the material. In a second, an individual was said to have developed such symptoms, and to have been hospitalized, for taking an undisclosed amount of kernels. None of the precise details as to the hows and whens of ingestion were available.

The two cases developed as the market for apricot and peach kernels was expanding rapidly across the country. Peach kernels, which have as high a concentration of vitamin B-17 (about 2 percent per kernel), were becoming almost as popular as apricot kernels, but the powers that be had not yet moved against the nation's peach crop.

The two new California cases served as the legal excuse for a series of outrageous actions by federal officials in several states, as they began threatening health food operators who dared to stock these natural food products. In 1976 in Florida, for example, federal agents raided a health food warehouse and confiscated 470 pounds of apricot kernels by asserting that they contained "a dangerous substance."

A U.S. attorney was quoted as saying that "the FDA has determined that 50 of the kernels eaten at once could be fatal to an adult and less would be fatal to a child."

We have no idea how any such determination was reached — and it is certainly news to the Hunzakuts, who may consume twice that number in any given day — and even to the Pueblo Indians of the Southwestern U.S.A. who used to prepare a brew made of the kernels of cherries, apricots, peaches and other substances containing B-17, while reportedly maintaining a low level of cancer incidence.

As to 50 kernels "eaten all at once" — here indeed was a puzzler. The human gullet simply cannot take 50 apricot kernels "all at once."

But no matter. The campaign against apricot kernels was on, following the campaign against Aprikern and Bee Seventeen. B-17 enthusiasts wondered if the Feds would turn next to the seeds of peaches, plums, pears, prunes, and nectarines, or even clamp down on blackberries.

It is of course possible to eat too much of anything at any given time. A thimbleful of water is toxic if injected into the lung; a bubble of air is fatal if injected into the bloodstream. That some people may have allergic reactions to apricot seeds (or anything else), or that a child may consume "too many," or that even an adult, taking leave of his rational biological senses, may consume a pound or two of seeds, is of course possible.

Too, those populations with high incidence of foods containing Vitamin B-17 are usually aware that they should not "overdo." In the Philippines, for example, the author found that Filipinos still eating the basic hinterland diet, which includes much cassava in various forms, are aware of the toxic reactions that come from overeating — or cooking — bitter cassava. These people, however, do what biological reason tells them to do when approaching a possible toxic reaction from their natural foods: They temporarily stop eating them.

In the meantime, Genesis 1:29 reminds us that God "has given you ... every tree with seed in its fruit; you shall have them for food."

CHAPTER NINE

That Astounding Vitamin: B-17

BY THE SUMMER OF 1973, with news breaking simultaneously on several fronts, the media again began to take notice of Laetrile — but this time in conjunction with a host of concerns and fads popularized by the return-to-nature craze. Nutritional approaches to health and medicine and belief in the superior value of whole foods were not new, of course; but when coupled with the fresh interest in vitamins and "natural" approaches to therapy, they tended to take on a new dimension. Laetrile, the "natural" answer to cancer, became part of the scenario. Hence the significant, if amusing, coalition of counterculture enthusiasts and the more traditional, even conservative, supporters of the substance.

It was perhaps the readiness of antiestablishmentarians to lump vitamin B-17 in with everything else of a seemingly unorthodox approach in the fight for good health that led Ernst Krebs, Jr., addressing that summer's Los Angeles conference on nontoxic cancer remedies, to warn of "heresy" — that is, departure from the strict Laetrile line in dealing with cancer. I had come to know and appreciate the intellect of this San Francisco scientist over the several years I was involved in the Laetrile story, and I was fully aware that in his mind Laetrile and indeed the whole question of cancer took on an almost religious significance. Krebs remains the most forthright, convinced exponent of the Beardian theory and champion of the vitamin-deficiency nature of cancer.

At his San Francisco mansion during one of the many memorable interviews in which this voluble savant spoke nonstop on the theory, nature, and solution of cancer, he said: "Laetrile needs true-believers — men moving ahead unequivocally toward a single goal." But he cautioned: "Remember, cancer is the last bastion of religious thinking — and anything is phony that won't stand the examination of a six-year-old boy." This was his way of summing up what he considers to be the illogical thinking of orthodox science in treating the cancer problem, one which he sees as basically simple, whose solution is found in the "universality of things."

FREEDOM FROM CANCER

The biochemist who taught himself several languages in order to read every extant document about amygdalin and the pancreatic enzymes approach to cancer has difficulty in articulating, for the layman, not only the specifics of Laetrile therapy but the mental motivation behind its discovery and use. But he took special pains to put forward his point of view to me, and it ran this way:

"The most open-minded, free-wheeling soul in the world will go up the wall if you tell him cancer is a specific vitamin-deficiency disease. And it took us thirteen years to realize that Laetrile is a new vitamin — B-17.

"So much a part of our thinking is that cancer represents a cell that must be killed. How can something nontoxic affect a malignant cell? To date, our cancer approach has been a drug approach — kill it, cut it, blast it out.

"What we are saying is that Laetrile is an anti-neoplastic vitamin, that vitamins are part of the universality. The mind has a psychological incapacity to determine how cancer can be caused not *by* something but by a *lack* of something, in this case, vitamin B-17."

Krebs, Jr. spent much of the 1960s elaborating the vitamin approach to Laetrile and cancer, and how they relate to enzymes, prevention and "control." He explained that the "first line of defense" against cancer is an intrinsic factor — "the totality of the pancreatic enzymes" and supporting immunological system of the body. These systems are influenced by vitamins and diet in how they operate. Processed foods, particularly refined sugar, play a role in weakening these systems, he asserted. The "second line of defense," which becomes the primary one when the "first line of defense" is weakened, constitutes the extrinsic factor, what Krebs calls vitamin B-17, "the surveillant anti-neoplastic vitamin."

I asked him several times if, in his view, he believed that a sufficient quantity of the "extrinsic factor" would work to prevent cancer even though the "intrinsic factor" — again, the enzymes and immunological system — continued to be weakened and an individual compounded the problem by persisting in noxious habits, say, smoking.

Yes, said the biochemist, "clinical cancer" would probably be prevented with enough vitamin B-17. That does not mean a person would *not* have cancer, which, if the Beardian theory holds true, is simply the appearance of trophoblast in the wrong place at the wrong time. What it means is that even if cancer developed time and again, the "second line of defense" — the nitriloside (Laetrile, amygdalin, vitamin B-17) — would be doing its job in continually inhibiting tumor growth. Hence his view that cancer is at root a vitamin-deficiency disease — both in the way the totality of vitamins and diet affect the pancreatic enzymes and the immunological mechanism and in the way removal of a natural-food factor from Western diets by food refining and processing has left the body virtually defenseless against the proliferation of cancer.

If the premise is ceded that cancer, like scurvy, rickets, pellagra, beriberi, and pernicious anemia, is a vitamin-deficiency disease, the next step is to demonstrate it. Krebs' extensive research points to Western "progress in agriculture and food processing as the primary culprit in the cancer picture, for it has removed vitamin B-17 in substantial amounts from the food we eat." He noted that a primary source of vitamin B-17 is millet. "Yet we abandoned millet and went on to wheat. And we quit eating the seeds of common fruits as our affluence grew."

In unison with the natural-foods school, Krebs notes that animals instinctively consume whole fruits and seeds — and also instinctively turn to the natural plants and grasses they need when they feel ill. This has been demonstrated by several veterinarians who, by 1976, had noted some success with retarding cancer in domesticated cats and dogs.

Where does one get vitamin B-17?

Krebs has kept an updated list of sources, since as the preventive aspects of Laetrile have tended to overshadow in importance its therapeutic aspects, the reliance on a B-17-laden diet becomes paramount.

As the San Franciscan told audiences around the country, sufficient intake of B-17 is a virtual guarantee that no clinical cancer will ever occur. The seeds of all fruits (except citrus fruits) grown in North America contain B-17, he points out, but the most abundant sources are peach and apricot kernels (where B-17 in concentrations as high as 2 percent is present) and in cherry seeds. The seeds of nectarines, pears, plums and prunes are likewise high in the substance.

Among beans, the broad beans (*Vicia faba*), burma, garbanzos or chickpeas, lentils (sprouted), mung (sprouted), lima, Rangoon and scarlet runner all contain nitriloside. Among nuts, the bitter almond (which is available in Eruope but is not generally available in the U.S.) contains perhaps the highest single concentration of B-17; the sweet almond no longer contains B-17; macadamias and cashews both do. Almost all wild berries contain B-17, very much including blackberries, chokeberries, Christmas berries, cranberries, elderberries, raspberries and strawberries. Among seeds: chia, flax, sesame. Among grains: oat groats, barley, brown rice (unpolished wild rice), buckwheat groats, chia, flax, millet, rye, vetch, wheat berries. Among grasses: acacia, alfalfa (sprouted), aquatic, Johnson, milkweed, Sudan, tunus, velvet, wheat grass, and white clover. Other good sources include cassava (also known as manioc or yucca), bamboo shoots, fuschia plant, sorghum, wild hydrangea, and the needles and fresh leaves of the yew tree.

The manufactured vitamin B-17, or the purified extract of amygdalin, is usually taken from apricot kernels by a process already discussed. Obviously, ways to synthesize Laetrile or extract it from even more abundant sources would lead to a more inexpensive, more easily accessible product.

While the modern experience of the Hunza people tends to bolster the natural-food approach to medicine in general, and the considerable consumption of apricots by those people tends to support the Laetrile theory in particular, Krebs has assembled a considerable backlog of data to underscore these premises:

1. Cancer is essentially a disease of civilization — that is, its incidence is high in the allegedly "civilized" countries, and diminishes as people decline on the "civilization" scale.

2. The primary variable in "uncivilized" habits is diet.

3. In the case of cancer, we are dealing with a specific vitamin-deficiency disease, and the specific deficiency is of vitamin B-17.

Krebs is fond of pointing to the fascinating data assembled by Vilhjalmur Stefansson in *Cancer: Disease of Civilization*, which appeared in 1960 and was a compilation of data on "primitive" peoples of both hemispheres to support the theory that cancer and diet are somehow linked. The writer did not leap to the nitriloside conclusion, but he left a large door open to it. A search of the documentation of missionaries, whalers, explorers, and government agents in Alaska led Stefansson to report that cancer was simply unknown among "uncivilized Eskimos" at the turn of the century, and that incidents of it did not even show up until into the third decade. Indeed, he reported, the Prudential Insurance Company of New York stated as fact in 1915 that "uncivilized people (such as the Canadian Eskimos) have little or no cancer." This statement produced no wonderment in 1915. Yet in 1956, such a statistic startled practically everybody when the *Canadian Medical Association Journal* reported it, he wrote. He quoted a U.S. War Department *Arctic Manual* statement in 1940: "Cancer has not yet been reported from uncivilized Eskimos."[1]

It intrigued Stefansson and medical researchers that the Eskimos had a very meaty and vegetable-deficient diet. Yet, they noted, such "primitives" as the Hunzakuts had a very vegetable-prone diet with minimal meat intake. But both were essentially cancer-free. Hence, the question of vegetarianism versus meat consumption did not seem to arise regarding cancer.

For Dr. Krebs, the difference is irrelevant. What is important, he believes, is the nitriloside-rich grasses consumed by the animals that the Eskimos eat; and the nitriloside-rich fruits and seeds — most particularly apricots — that the Hunzas consume.

In a John Beard Memorial Foundation memorandum to the

National Cancer Institute's Dr. Dean Burk, Dr. Krebs referred to a United Press summary (February 1949) of a five-author paper in the *Journal of the American Medical Association* on why there are so few cases of cancer among Hopi and Navajo Indians. The memo read in part: "The Indians' diet seems to be low in quality and quantity and wanting in variety and the doctors wondered if this had anything to do with the fact that only 36 cases of malignant cancer were found out of 30,000 admissions to Ganado, Arizona, Mission Hospital.

"In the same population of white persons, the doctor said there would have been about 1,800."

Concluded Krebs: "In the Navajos there were 36 cases of cancer where there should have been 1,800 — or only 2 percent of the expected number. At the time of this study, the incidence of cancer in rural white populations as compared to urban ones was 70 percent.

"The rural white population had a 'better' or larger and more calorific diet. It differed from the Indian population in lacking the vitamin B-17 or nitriloside found in the diet of the Indian population."

Both Krebs and other researchers have looked at studies of the Nigerian population in which a high consumption of cassava is paralleled not only by much lower rates of cancer but also by apparent control of the "hemolytic crisis" of sickle-cell anemia.

Cassava as a staple among Filipinos in connection with much lower rates of cancer in the Filipino countryside was observed by this author in visits to that country between 1971 and 1975. Indeed, as in all so-called "primitive" diets, the intake of highly nitrilosidic foods, the use of whole, natural foods, and less reliance on animal proteins is apparently linked with natural longevity and much lower incidences of the degenerative (in contrast to the infectious or parasitic) diseases.

I found veterans of the Huk movement and other natives of Luzon living well into their 80s and 90s on the same diet they had enjoyed for years — cassava (including "cassava cakes"), unpolished wild rice, black beans, *camote* tops, and many grasses and vegetables either known to be, or suspect of being, nitrilosidic.

The diet of the Ilocano Filipinos is particularly striking — mostly vegetarian and including a host of plants and vegetables, a special delicacy is *papait* ("bitter"), which consists of partially digested plant material in the digestive tracts of goats. The "bitter" is probably as nitrilosidic as the concoction of "primitive Eskimos," consisting of partially digested and highly nitrilosidic tundra grass from the rumen of caribou and laced with seal oil.

In the summer of 1975 I inquired of Tausog Muslim refugees from Jolo Island, Philippines, about their staple diet. Intriguingly enough, I had to pass through a battery of interpreters (English to Tagalog, Tagalog to Chabacano, Chabacano to Tausog) in order to learn that yes, cassava is the staple among the Jolo Muslims and that, yes, cancer is virtually unknown there. When the word "cancer" was finally explained to the elderly lady with whom I was speaking, she responded — and this was translated back "up" through the four languages or dialects — that "eaters of beef and pork" (her gentle way to say "Christians") were known to come down with the disease on Jolo, but for the basic population cancer was virtually unknown.

Natural whole foods, less animal protein and higher nitrilosidic intake are common among such longevity-famous peoples as the Abkhasians of the Soviet Union and the amazing Vilcabamba Indians of Ecuador, who also reflect virtually none of the "killer diseases" of civilization — arteriosclerosis, heart disease, or cancer.

In 1975, Doctors Mas Goenawan and Todotua Simandjuntak of Indonesia revealed their longtime work in cancer therapy with 6,000 patients at the Cisarua Health Resort in Bogor, Indonesia. The treatments, all of them showing positive benefit, were done with the leaves of, baths in, or poultices made from bitter cassava. This particular B-17-containing therapy led the medics to conclude that the cassava itself should be preventative as well as therapeutic in dealing with cancer, that radiation and chemotherapy, which they also used, do themselves cause cancer and that patients who received *only* the cassava therapy and had never undergone "orthodox" treatment responded better.

In a paper prepared for the McNaughton Foundation and researching nitriloside consumption by man and animals, Krebs called attention to the "relative freedom of wild and most domestic herbivores from cancer as contrasted to its higher incidence among at least domesticated carnivores." A spectacular case in point, he said, was the cancer incidence among bears in the San Diego Zoo. He claimed five had died in one grotto there in the last six years — all of cancer of the liver and all after having been given "a diet almost completely free from nitrilosides."[2]

The nitriloside content of pasturage, fodder, and silage is "often striking," he said, noting as "common and often rich sources of nitrilosides" white clover, alfalfa or lucerne, vetch, certain millets, Johnson grass, Sudan grass, Arrow grass, the various sorghums, lupines, broad beans, velvet grass, and at least eight other grasses, and the leaves of *Rosacae* and berries. Indeed, the two most common of the pasture grasses, Johnson and Sudan, often carry as much as 15,000 to 20,000 milligrams of nitriloside per kilogram of dry grass, thus offering a diet spectacularly heavier in vitamin B-17 than that available to *Homo sapiens*, he said. Krebs called the incidence of cancer in domesticated horses "reasonably high, though no formal statistics are obviously available."

Krebs has little patience with opposing views on the cause, nature, and control of cancer. In one of our interviews, he said: "Look, there is the highest increase in cancer in the history of mankind. If it continues it alone will take care of the so-called population explosion. There is an identical growth rate in cancer all around the Western world — and those places where Western nutrition has gone."

Defending the view that "cancer represents a local manifestation of a systemic disease," and that viruses and poisons, however much they may "organize" cancer, by no means "cause" it, Krebs described the action of Laetrile as a magnet aimed at pulling out metal pellets embedded in the body. "Just assume the body is loaded with these pellets, which may be anywhere. Along comes a magnet to pull them out. According to where the pellets are in the body, the patient will die, or improve, or recover from the process." Hence the explanation for dead Laetrile patients as well as living and only partly recovered ones, he said.

The ever-recurring question on my mind to all concerned in the Laetrile battle was this: If there is evidence, even fragmentary evidence, of at least partial efficacy through use of Laetrile, then why the obvious suppression of it?

"The anti-Laetrile campaign seems to be inspired by sheer, naked terror, for Laetrile represents the most terrifying possibility in medicine — a time when we could no longer say of cancer, 'we'd better go in there and cut it out,' " said Krebs, who exhibits most emotion when explaining why his has been an uphill battle. The *creme de la creme* of medicine is surgery, said Laetrile's pioneer. Surgery would be dealt a setback if it became commonly known that the solution to cancer is diet, not the surgeon's knife.

"The U.S.A. has more moron factories — the universities — than anywhere else in the world," he said, criticizing a seeming disinterest on campuses in looking into the dietary approach to cancer. He termed the American Medical Association and Food and Drug Administration "closed systems — blind, unconscious, but not consciously evil. If we were making progress in cancer why is one person out of three dying from it? If you bring in Laetrile you've eliminated the department of tissue pathology, therapeutic radiology, and will have made one hell of a dent into surgery." Both "billions of dollars at stake" in cancer therapy as presently practiced and "fantastic ego considerations" of scientists and bureaucrats committed to a faulty premise are at the root of the attack against Laetrile, he believes.

The "chief harassment" against him in California came not so much from the FDA itself as from the State Department of Public Health. But nationwide it was the FDA that remained "on the trail" of Laetrile movements across state lines. The FDA, he believes, is strongly influenced by lobbying groups such as the AMA, American Cancer Society, and the producers and suppliers of X-ray equipment and the officially okayed anticancer drugs. The FDA represents a bureaucratic implementation of these pressures, he believes.

Notwithstanding the climate of hostility, the student who turned from medicine to biochemistry and physiology has put together a "Laetrile team" — between 125 and 150 noncancerous people from around the world who are regularly using Laetrile to provide support for his contention that enough daily intake of B-17 acts as a preventative against cancer. "They have never developed cancer — not one. Naturally, if they did, the whole thing would collapse," he said.

The outspoken doctor has estimated that such peoples as the Hunzakuts, "primitive" Eskimos, certain African and South American tribes, Australian aborigines and the North American Indians in their native state consume diets carrying anywhere from 250 to 3,000 mg. of nitriloside per day, while "civilized" man relies on a diet certainly providing no more than 2 percent of that amount, and in some cases far less.

There is, of course, no established "minimum daily requirement" of B-17, and by 1976 no binding answer could be given to the increasingly persistent questions of "how much B-17 — how many apricot or kernel seeds — do I need daily to stay cancer-free?" A general rule of thumb that was advanced is one apricot or peach kernel per 10 pounds of body weight, but this is not a definitive statement. All that can be reasonably ascertained is the strong parallel between obviously high concentrations of vitamin B-17 (amygdalin and its near-compounds) in the diet and obviously low incidences of degenerative diseases of all kinds, particularly cancer.

In the 1970s, Ernst Krebs, Jr. was far more assertive about the values of natural B-17 in the diet as the way to prevent cancer than he was in the constant controversy over the therapeutic use of vitamin B-17 as the product Laetrile. He also prepared menus which, he postulates, could maintain a probable preventative level of B-17 in the body's system.[3]

Aside from his fisticuffs with the FDA over bureaucracy, regulations, and licensing, Ernst Krebs, Jr. has also fought a holding action over another substance he and his father pioneered: pangametin, or pangamic acid, which he baptized vitamin B-15, an accessory food factor. In 1973, this item remained in a bureaucratic limbo imposed by the FDA in the United States, yet it was being extolled in the Soviet Union as a breakthrough in medicine.

In June and July, the *Journal of the American Medical Association* twice reported on Soviet successes with the substance, which was developed, championed, and revealed to the world by the Krebses. In the

July 23, 1973, *Journal,* it was noted that "another vitamin, synthesized by Prof. (Vasili) Bukin earlier, is vitamin B-15; this chemical entity aids in stimulating oxidative processes and energy exchange. It aids in delaying development of atherosclerosis in the aging individual, says Dr. Bukin." It was, of course, not Prof. Bukin who developed the vitamin, but the Krebses; Krebs, Jr. has come to believe the Biblical aphorism that a prophet is without honor in his own country.

In the matter of vitamin B-17 (Laetrile, nitriloside) Krebs has emphasized the *natural* approach to cancer. He told the San Francisco Vegetarian Society for Health and Humanity in January 1974: "We look forward to the time when we won't have Laetrile as such. We will rely upon foods rich in vitamin B-17 and the medical use of the material will no longer be necessary."

To the audience of vegetarians and natural-food champions, Krebs delivered the composite vitamin B-17 philosophy: The process of regeneration is natural and normal to the animal organism. The trophoblast, be it uterine or extragenital, is a natural part of the life cycle and it is naturally inhibited within that cycle. Vitamin B-17 is the naturally selected controlling, extrinsic antitrophoblastic factor, and the environment in which primitive man flourished was rich in vitamin B-17-containing foods. He turned to these foods for a variety of reasons just as sick animals today spontaneously seek out vitamin B-17-bearing grasses.

The reason why cancer has not been bred out of the human race through evolution, the biochemist told his audience, is that everyone develops cancer in the course of his life many times but it does not come to the clinical level because the intrinsic elements — the pancreatic enzymes and immunological system — are functioning.

He warned his audience about the "delusions of returning to nature by eating whole wheat or grains only, as they are deficient in vitamin B-17." Harvesting and cooking grains are, relatively speaking, only recent developments in man's history — of the two to three million years of the evolution of the presumptive primate stem from which man springs, "it has only been about 6,000 years that man has ceased getting his vitamin B-17 from the sprouts rather than from dried lima or dried mung beans. Man's forebears were getting concentrations of vitamin B-17 eight to ten times greater on the basis of the weight of the original food than we get," he said.

For one gram of dried mung beans, the modern human receives perhaps only one percent of the vitamin B-17 that man's forebears received when they ate such beans in the sprouting stage, Krebs pointed out. He went on to state that this is one reason for the fulminating dietary deficiency across the board. It is the height of human egotism, he contended, to assume that the culture of civilization, in a few thousand years, has built in the answer to the problems of deficiency that affect the living machinery. "We have had this profound deviation from biological experience and we're suffering the consequences of it, and when you return to sprouting, you go in the direction of correcting the consequences of this aberration," Krebs insisted.

"We are well advised to eat as broad a spectrum of vegetable food as we possibly can, to eat it as fresh as we can get it, to eat it in its sprouting state if we can get it, and above all, to eat it whole. And if we do that then we are infallible nutritionally, then we can say the Food and Drug Administration is correct when it says that the normal diet requires no supplementation. That would be the normal diet and it would not require supplementation."

Officialdom and orthodoxy, of course, have not yet accepted either amygdalin or the beta-cyanogenetic glucosides as a vitamin, or vitamins. Further, there is some confusion because Krebs considers the full range of beta-cyanogenetic glucosides to be vitamin B-17, while the McNaughton Foundation exclusively refers to amygdalin as B-17. At least one research report within California health department circles when this was written attacked the concept that the substance Laetrile is a vitamin. If Krebs' massive research on nitriloside is anywhere near the mark, then plainly nitriloside is a vitamin, meeting the usual definition that a vitamin is any of a group of constituents of most foods in their natural state, of which very small quantities are essential for the normal nutrition of animals.

A letter of December 18, 1973, to National Health Federation legislative advocate Clinton Miller from the "division of regulatory guidance, office of compliance, bureau of foods," FDA, bore a succinct message: "We have not officially defined the term vitamin."

In 1975, medical orthodoxy widely disseminated a direct attack on the presumptive vitamin nature of Laetrile by veteran biochemist David M. Greenberg, Ph. D.,[4] which mainly attacked Laetrile on the basis of Krebs' proposed local-action theory (the relevance of which to whether Laetrile "works" has already been demonstrated as minimal), but also claimed the beta-cyanogenetic glycosides do not fulfill the general requirements for classification as vitamins. However, the arguments were ranged around a denial of evidence, variously adduced in several quarters yet summarily dismissed by the author with ironclad finality. "No evidence has ever been adduced . . ." was the usual attack on the properties claimed for Laetrile.

The article must fairly be contrasted with Dr. Dean Burk's monograph released the same year[5] which makes an equally definitive case *for* the classification of amygdalin as Vitamin B-17. That both biochemists,

Burk being the then-retired chief of the cytochemistry division, National Cancer Institute, could reach diametrically opposed conclusions as to the vitamin nature of Laetrile reflects how inconclusive the debate may continue to be.

Dr. Krebs describes vitamin B-17 in its pure form as a white, sugary, slightly bitter crystalline substance which, like all other members of the B-vitamin complex and like all other water-soluble vitamins, is without toxicity. In fact, he said, when administered to diabetics, the quantities may be very large without any untoward effect whereas a comparable quantity of table sugar could be fatal.

In his speeches around the nation, Krebs said that Laetrile, in addition to its alleged anticancer properties, has a host of collateral biological or physiological functions including the production of benzoic acid, itself a detoxicant and containing antirheumatic properties. A breakdown product of vitamin B-17 is thiocyanate, which, among other things, has an action that reduces excessively high blood pressure.

The various metabolic uses of vitamin B-17 were, of course, key to the case of Dr. John A. Richardson in California, arrested on "cancer quackery" charges for allegedly dispensing Laetrile in the treatment of cancer. The state's health code recognized the use of amygdalin (again, the common and accepted chemical name for Laetrile or vitamin B-17) in treating metabolic deficiencies. The state statutes opposed its use solely in cancer treatment. The intriguing legal point remained: If a physician is simply treating the metabolism with vitamin therapy, it is surely legal to use vitamin B-17 even if the patient happens to have cancer. That the state took a dim view of this approach, which literally sidestepped all efforts at the crackdown against Laetrile, was the probable key motivation behind the doctor's continuing litigation.

What might turn out to be an almost equally impressive use of vitamin B-17 is the alleged prevention of the "hemolytic crisis" or severe symptoms of sickle-cell anemia. This possibility, of immediate importance to at least 50,000 American Negroes in the U.S. estimated to have the genetic sickle-cell trait, is just now being explored. A single research paper by Robert G. Houston of the Foundation for Mind Research, Pomona, N.Y., and drawing on some forty varying medical and scientific sources, reached a conclusion which warmed the cockles of Ernst Krebs, Jr.'s heart: The rarity of sickle-cell anemia in African Negroes as compared with those in the United States "is associated with a prevalence of thiocyanate-yielding foods in native African diets."[6] That is, cyanate, which the author terms an inhibitor of sickling (a defense Mother Nature may have supplied as a protection against malaria), develops from the oxidation of thiocyanate, which is formed from nitrilosides (the beta-cyanogenetic glucosides) in food plants. Here again, Dr. Krebs insists, we can see vitamin B-17 at work.

Concluded Houston: "Clinical use of cyanate and thiocyanate has ameliorated sickle-cell anemia at dosage levels derivable from African diets. It is proposed that the disease represents an unrelieved nutritional dependency on thiocyanate and nitriloside in those genetically affected." He referred to clinical trials at Rockefeller University as reported in 1972 by Gillette *et. al.* and a host of related studies.[7]

The underlying theory is this: the natural, vitamin B-17-containing foods in the African diet provide the extrinsic factor to the development of sickle-cell anemia among Negroes with the sickling trait. But no such extrinsic defense against the development of sickle-cell anemia among those with the sickling trait exists for American Negroes — who, by and large, are eating the same vitamin B-17-deficient processed foods as other Americans.

A San Francisco physician, Dr. Dennis Myers, began working in 1973 with sickle-cell anemia-afflicted black children, and by April 1974 was able to pinpoint an apparent case of sickle-cell anemia control of an eleven-year-old girl through the simple expedient of having her take oral doses of Laetrile on alternate days. She had been free of the need for hospitalization for almost eighteen months, he said. He added that he suspects a low, but still undetermined, level of nitriloside available from natural sources in seeds, kernels, and various foods is the best way to prevent the hemolytic crisis from developing.

Other claimed benefits made for vitamin B-17 in the diet, and as tabulated by Dr. Stewart Jones,[8] include help in prevention of pernicious anemia, amelioration of hypertension, and amelioration of arthritis symptoms.

Were vitamin B-17 to be a natural preventative of sickle-cell anemia as well as of cancer — or, if only helpful in both these areas — its two-in-one efficacy would make it the most potent vitamin known to man and its use one of the most astounding developments in modern science.

CHAPTER TEN

From Manila to Palo Alto:
Laetrile's Defenders

DETERMINED TO LEARN ALL I COULD about Laetrile, I sought out practitioners who had been in the forefront of the controversy since its beginning, and others who had just joined the battle. I wanted to know if those who had been impressed by the early Laetrile results were still interested, or if they now believed the Laetrile approach was in error.

It was therefore fascinating to me to note the similarity of views between one of the Laetrile pioneers, Dr. Manuel Navarro of the Philippines, a committed Laetrile therapist since the 1950s and a key developer of the urine test for detection of cancer, and Dr. Stewart M. Jones, Palo Alto, California, who recently turned from skeptic to convinced laetrilist and outspoken opponent of the medical bureaucracy. For Dr. Jones, there was a personal stake: his mother was suffering from tongue cancer, and he found Laetrile of positive benefit. For Dr. Navarro, Laetrile has been a labor of love for two decades. For Dr. Jones, the use of Laetrile had meant a pitched battle since 1971.

Dr. Navarro, the primary Asian advocate of the unitarian or trophoblastic theory of cancer and the use of Laetrile in cancer therapy, has been battling on the side of Laetrile efficacy in word and deed for well over twenty years. While on a news-gathering tour of Southeast Asia in August-September 1973, I met the wiry, soft-spoken, longtime scientist at his office in the University of Santo Tomas in Manila, and had followup interviews in 1974 and 1975.

Although he has worked with Laetrile since the information on it became known worldwide in the 1950s, the professor of medicine and surgery had dealt with about 1,000 cases personally at the time of our interview; he was still dependent on Mexico for supplies of the substance. But of those 1,000 cases, he told me, ninety-five percent showed "positive signs of relief, particularly relief of pain" and even during the early days of 100-milligram doses this palliative effect was noticeable. Dr. Navarro has since upped the active dosage to as high as fourteen grams per day in some cases.

A faithful adherent of the unitarian theory, Dr. Navarro developed a refined test for detection of human chorionic gonadotropin (HCG) in cancer patients in 1963 at the University of Santo Tomas. He came up with the test by utilizing a similar approach for the detection of pregnancies.

That both cancer patients and pregnant women secrete the HCG hormone, quite in keeping with unitarian theory, has been accepted by some of Laetrile's opponents, even though the "UT" theory overall — as the earlier Beard Anthrone Test (BAT) — has been denounced by state departments of public health. Navarro and his associates utilized the immunological test for cancer detection and, as late as 1971, had detected HCG in the urine of 1,563 cases of proven cancer located from head to foot and belonging to thirty-four different histological types. Included were cases of leukemia.[1]

Navarro argued repeatedly in medical journals that the HCG "immunoassay" usable in detecting pregnancies could also be utilized for the early detection of cancer while it is still amenable to treatment or to protect against postoperative recurrence. "I had been laughed at for using the urine test, but now it is being used in America," Navarro told me with a wink. He referred to the 1969 report of J. E. Dailey and P. M. Marcuse, who noted: "Detection of chorionic gonadotropin may be an aid in the diagnosis of bronchogenic carcinoma (lung cancer) . . . . A positive test for chorionic gonadotropin in the urine is confirmatory evidence of a gonadotropin-producing tumor. The use of more sensitive techniques such as the hemagglutination test for chorionic gonadotropin might lead to the diagnosis of more patients with bronchogenic carcinoma while they are still amenable to treatment."[2]

This was even before Dr. Navarro was aware of the Braunstein study in July 1973, which helped put the frosting on the cake. Using modern radio-immunoassay techniques for examining serum, Braunstein and his associates reported the presence of the hormone in a substantial number of patients with a variety of tumors.[3]

The California Cancer Advisory Council's attack on the earlier BAT (Beard Anthrone Test) in 1964 had found that the test was "of no value in the diagnosis of cancer." It added: "The Cancer Advisory Council hereby recommends to the State Department of Public Health that all persons, firms, associations and other entities administering the said anthrone test or one substantially similar thereto as a diagnostic agent for cancer, be ordered to cease and desist from such administering, and that appropriate proceedings be taken to give immediate effect to this recommendation."[4]

The laetrilists would argue that it would behoove American science to reexamine the urine test for cancer detection, a method routinely used by Doctors Contreras and Richardson.

The reality that both pregnant women and cancer patients would secrete HCG follows from the unitarian thesis, and as late as 1972 more orthodox journals were coming close to a recognition of the similarity between cancer and the embroyological process. For example, in *Science* for October 17, 1972, pathologist D. H. Koobs concluded an article with these interesting observations: "Perhaps carcinogens, including viruses, uproot the control mechanisms normally associated with the program of conception. Because cancer cell metabolism and growth characteristics are so similar to the process of conception, it appears that the immunologic manipulation which allows the maternal host first to tolerate — then reject — the physiologic 'tumor' is indeed a good model for investigating cancer therapy."[5] Particularly, this layman might add, if the Beard premise — that cancer and trophoblast are the same thing — is true.

Hence, it follows that HCG is secreted in "natural" pregnancy and "unnatural" cancer, if the unitarian or trophoblastic theory of cancer — that the trophoblast in pregnancy and cancer are the same thing — is correct, or even mostly correct. A company that manufactures pregnancy testing kits "simply cannot understand why a pregnancy test it has devised can be used for detecting cancer," Navarro said in Manila. He remains as outspoken as Krebs in trying to explain the entrenched opposition to Laetrile, let alone the opposition to the "UT" approach to diagnosis.

"It's economics," he told me. "The surgeons will lose patients, the radiologists will lose patients, X-ray machine makers will be affected, drug companies manufacturing cancer drugs will be affected. Aspirin itself and other pain killers will be affected." The Laetrile theory and use are just too simple to be easily accepted by medical orthodoxy, he argued, noting that his own battle in the Philippines has been waged against a medical establishment profoundly influenced by the Americans.

A similar case is made by Palo Alto's angry Dr. Stewart M. Jones, who was incensed enough about what he found to be loaded arguments against Laetrile without much supportive data that he investigated the matter thoroughly. The product of his investigation, ultimately, was his own booklet, *Nutrition Rudiments in Cancer*, distributed in 1972 by the Committee for Freedom of Choice in Cancer Therapy. It provided the stimulus for heated debate between Dr. Jones and fellow physicians.

Dr. Jones states boldly and bluntly:

> *The cancer industry in the U.S.A. has become so large and its beneficiaries so powerful, that any truly promising prophylaxis and control of cancer is bound to encounter powerful resistance. Many before Laetrile have been squelched by such measures as the ACS' Ca-A Jour-*

nal for Clinicians *under the "Unproven Methods of Cancer Management," or by the FDA.*

Articles favorable to measures banned by the FDA, AMA and ACS are regularly shunned by scientific journals in the U.S.A. because of the fear of loss of status if such topics are covered. This reticence of scientific journals to publish such politically controversial material leads to widespread ignorance among M.D.'s about Laetrile and other methods.

Scientific rationale and clinical results are not factors influencing the acceptance of a promising prophylaxis and control of cancer except in an inverse way. The more promising such a method appears, the more strenuously do the beneficiaries of the entrenched cancer industry and their agents rationalize, malign, exaggerate and otherwise obfuscate against the facts about the proposed method.

Students of Laetrile and banned vitamins B-15 and B-17 are relatively weak, as individuals, in any fight against the entrenched, united economic beneficiaries of the cancer industry. They should leave such a fight to the entrenched, economic beneficiaries of any successful prophylaxis and cure of cancer — such as the mammoth life insurance and medical insurance companies — when they awaken from slumber.

Moreover, wrote Dr. Jones:

This huge industry provides life-sustaining revenues and desirable standards of living and social position to the following groups of people (a partial list):

Surgeons who do cancer surgery, oncologists and other internists, general practitioners who treat cancer victims, gynecologists, pediatricians treating cancer in children, nurses who treat and care for cancer victims, all research scientists engaging in cancer research, all employees and stockholders of the following: nursing homes, hospitals, radiation equipment manufacturers and servicing organizations, therapeutic X-ray equipment makers, hospital suppliers, medical and surgical suppliers . . . .[6]

Dr. Jones first became involved in the Laetrile story when he read the attack on Laetrile in "Unproven Methods of Cancer Management" in *Cancer* (October 1971). The Palo Alto physician recalled that he had read enough attacks on Laetrile to reach the assumption that it must be truly dangerous. But when he went looking for documentation to "disprove" what the laetrilists were saying, he could find little. "The more I delved into it, the more incensed I became," he said. He read all that he could, including Howard Beard's massive work, and became convinced of the nutritional aspects of cancer in general and the efficacy of Laetrile in particular.

Unlike Dr. John Richardson from nearby Albany, Dr. Jones did not start treating cancer patients. He did, however, make arrangements to be able to "lend" Laetrile. "I do not sell or prescribe Laetrile. I lend it, and I only accept repayment in kind," he said, fully aware of California law. "You can lend anybody anything. I also tell people I am not treating their cancer — they are left under their own doctor's care. I do say I treat patients for nutritional needs, and this includes B-17. I advise against radiation and chemotherapy."

Since he became convinced about the efficacy of Laetrile, Dr. Jones reports, he "dealt with" fifty to sixty patients between 1971 and 1973. All of these, he now says, exhibited various kinds of relief, particularly in analgesic responses. He became so excited over the nutritional approach to cancer that he circulated his booklet to nearly 400 medical students at Stanford University Medical School and Research Center, as well as to every member of the San Mateo County Medical Society. But the early reaction was upsetting. It ranged, he recalled, "from mild interest to complete apathy."

Nonetheless, because of the widespread circulation of his views, Dr. Jones learned that far more people than he had ever supposed were in fact using Laetrile, availing themselves of the "Laetrile underground" in California or making the "Tijuana connection" in Mexico. He invited me to examine his copious files on Laetrile use, including correspondence from physicians. On the surface they tended to confirm the remark to me by Robert Bradford, President of the Committee for Freedom of Choice in Cancer Therapy, that some 800 physicians around the country were using Laetrile — whether they called it amygdalin, vitamin B-17, or nitriloside.

Wrote a Philadelphia M.D.: "Many thanks for the recent literature. I am using amygdalin personally and professionally but have not had sufficient time for complete evaluation."

Wrote a Honolulu nutritionist to a Burlingame, California, physician whose letter attacking Dr. Jones was published in *Cancer News Journal*:

> *I have personal experience with Laetrile and nutrition in the treatment of cancer. My own brother was stricken with Hodgkin's disease and given three months to live. That was over three years ago. A tumor in his chest was almost volleyball size and was completely dissolved after he underwent Laetrile treatment in Mexico and was put on a strict diet that included megavitamin therapy. He now golfs twice a week and took his family on a 5,000-mile road trip to celebrate his recovery. His is only one of many, many examples.*

Urged by another physician in California to turn over documents he had on Laetrile efficacy in cancer treatment — a request frequently pressed by the State Department of Public Health — Dr. Jones wrote in March 1973:

> ... *Nothing would delight me more than to review records of my cancer patients who have been under Laetrile therapy, with you or anyone else who may be interested.*
>
> *However, if I or you treated anyone who had cancer with laetrile, the United States Federal Drug Administration [sic] and the California Drug Administration [sic] would have long ago confiscated our records and arrested us. The fate of Doctor Richardson of Albany is certainly testimony to this fact . . . .*
>
> *There are many people in the Bay Area that showed improvement or arrest of their documented malignancies after Laetrile therapy. Some doctors in the California medical hierarchy are presently taking Laetrile for their own cancers. Most of the records of local patients who have or are receiving Laetrile therapy are with Doctor Contreras of Mexico or Doctor Hans Nieper of Germany.*
>
> *Any doctor treating them openly here is breaking the law. You certainly are aware of this, I am sure.*

Dr. Jones perceived his role as tilting at the windmill of entrenched medical orthodoxy and its overlap with economics any way he could. (Hence the preface to his booklet: "Dedicated to economics, which makes politics understandable and bedfellows less strange.") He took up the cudgels for eighty-six-year-old nutritionist Emory Thurston, who was arrested and released on $2,000 bail for "practicing medicine without a license" in supplying Laetrile, and for Dr. Harvey E. Howard, who was arrested after selling Laetrile to an undercover agent. In the first case, a supply of Dr. Jones' books was confiscated when Thurston, executive secretary of the Institute of Nutritional Research in Hollywood, was arrested. In the latter case, Jones wrote to the Chino Institution for Men in behalf of the incarcerated Dr. Howard:

> *I have been very much impressed with Dr. Howard's knowledge of nutrition and his dedication to helping anyone who needed help, especially persons suffering from cancer, who are the innocent victims of our vicious and discriminatory state law against the use of Laetrile for the treatment of cancer.*
>
> *I have personally seen dozens of cases of cancer, many of them poisoned or disfigured by the California state-allowed treatments of surgery, radiation or chemotherapy, that improved after taking Laetrile. Many of these patients, considered terminal by orthodox M.D.'s, had dramatic improvement even from the first dose of Laetrile . . . .*

> *Personally, I feel that the members of the Department of Public Health for the State of California, and the California FDA, Fraud Department, should be the ones jailed because of their inhuman, discriminatory laws against the victims of cancer who are forced to accept the state approved lethal treatments. Only California and Pennsylvania have these disgraceful laws which result in the arrest of someone like Dr. Howard who was entrapped by the unscrupulous agent ... while trying to help what he thought was a bona fide patient. At night before I go to sleep I often think of those miserable people who are bringing so much suffering to the cancer victims in order to preserve the huge cancer industry.*

Dr. Jones, by no means a John Bircher, is convinced of the conspiratorial nature of what he calls the "industrial-medical-government triumvirate" and says the individuals who compose it "are behaving just as rationally as most people everywhere have always behaved when choosing between secure maintenance of a comfortable economic status quo and severe economic sacrifice to promote the general welfare." (And, hence, the postscript to his booklet: "It is far more profitable to look for a cancer cure than to find one.")

There is a way, he suggests, to oppose "Laetrile suppression." As he writes in his booklet: "The effective way to oppose Laetrile suppression is to enlist and band together those interests which would economically benefit most by worldwide Laetrile prophylaxis of cancer. A partial list would include: life insurance companies, medical insurance companies, tobacco companies, cyclamate manufacturers, all manufacturers of carcinogenic substances, beef and poultry growers, makers of DES ...."

Such a union, he believes, would be an effective economic coalition against the coalition-by-convenience-or-design of medical orthodoxy, federal regulatory agencies, and the pharmaceutical industry.

Jones was, of course, forced to pay for his temerity.

As the State of California — the only state with specific anti-Laetrile legislation written into state codes — was losing its lengthy and costly misdemeanor trials against John A. Richardson, M.D., The Powers That Be fell back on the time-honored tactic of peer review:

Dr. Jones was called before the State Board of Medical Examiners in 1975 and variously accused of incompetence, making false statements, and moral turpitude because of his use of Laetrile (vitamin B-17) in therapy, even though he had carefully explained to one and all that he was using vitamin B-17 along with other vitamins, enzymes, minerals and dietary manipulation as part of nutritional or metabolic therapy.

The on-again, off-again hearings produced at least one happy result:

One of the physicians on the board resigned from the hearing because he uses Laetrile himself as a cancer patient and could hardly stomach the spectacle of sitting in judgment on a man accused of using an "unproven remedy" he had found beneficial in his own case.

Ultimately, Jones was exonerated of all but one loophole offense — violation of an amazing California Department of Public Health-California Administrative Code section which prohibits the prescription, sale or other distribution of Laetrile "to any patient who has or who *believes* [emphasis ours] he has cancer." Dr. Jones was placed on two years' probation; a one-year suspension of his medical license was stayed.

CHAPTER ELEVEN

An Insider's Battle:
Dean Burk at Work

"DOCTORS HAVE GONE THE OTHER ROUTE NOW — they're no longer opposed to Laetrile. They've seen their patients die like flies with traditional treatment and they've decided to give themselves and their families a better chance."

The speaker was Dean Burk, for years the lone, single voice within the federal government persistently arguing for a fair trial for Laetrile. This one-man movement was speaking to the *Anaheim Register*, January 22, 1973, on the fact that he knew that amygdalin — Laetrile's chemical or generic name — was in common use by doctors in cancer treatment, despite opposition to Laetrile by the Food and Drug Administration, the American Medical Association, and the American Cancer Society. Dean Burk could speak with unusual authority. As head of the cytochemistry section of the National Cancer Institute (NCI) and concerned with cancer research for forty-five years, the California-born researcher had been actively involved in Laetrile probes since 1968. He had become an outspoken champion not of the total efficacy of Laetrile, let alone of the unitarian thesis (which he frankly pooh-poohed, at least in part), but of the need for fair testing of the substance.

The salty, cigar-chomping, phrase-making biochemist usually took on, entirely alone, the National Cancer Institute, the FDA, and the medical bureaucracy itself, testifying before Congress on Laetrile, writing legislators, rebutting the official line whenever possible, speaking out publicly and risking condemnation from the ranks of government.

At NCI headquarters in Bethesda, Maryland, his colleagues took a dimmer view of his activities. As an NCI spokesman told the *Los Angeles Times*, July 16, 1973:

> *The NCI has consistently held the position that Dr. Burk has the right to exercise his freedom of speech if he makes it abundantly clear that he does so as a private citizen and not as a representative of the institute. However, as a result of inappropriate advocacy of Laetrile, Dr.*

Burk has been officially reprimanded for violations of the Department of Health, Education and Welfare's standards of official conduct.

To which Burk responded: "I love the National Cancer Institute and even helped to create it, but I don't like to see any public servant telling lies to the public. They did get some positive results (on Laetrile tests on mice), much to their surprise and disappointment."

By 1974, Burk, who never held the position that Laetrile was the single answer to cancer, was almost as enamored of the chemical hydrazine sulfate — making sudden, startling progress in tests on cancer control — as he had been of Laetrile.

The veteran biochemist, whose multi-degreed, merit-winning background takes up thirty lines in *Who's Who in the World,* began his interest in Laetrile by conducting tests on animals at the suggestion of the McNaughton Foundation's founder-president. These early results showed Burk there was "something" to Laetrile.

A thorough scientist who often told me he was keeping his mind open to every possibility about cancer (and everything else), Burk actually had associated himself more with Otto Warburg's thesis that the prime cause of cancer is the replacement of oxygen in normal body cells by a fermentation of sugar. Burk edited the English edition of Warburg's "The Prime Cause and Prevention of Cancer" lecture before Nobel laureates in 1966. Warburg's attack on the more "orthodox" concept that cancer is essentially a virus-caused disease remains among the more lucid putdowns of that concept. As translated by Dr. Burk:

> *To conclude the discussion on the prime cause of cancer, the virus theory of cancer may be mentioned. It is the most cherished topic of the philosophers of cancer. If it were true, it would be possible to prevent and cure cancer by the methods of virology; and all carcinogens could be eaten or smoked freely without any danger, if only contact with the cancer virus would be avoided.*

Two realities most disturbed the veteran biochemist during his battle with The Powers That Be: First, he knew (and said so in various public lectures entitled "A Very Grim Picture") that conventional, orthodox cancer drugs are toxic and that their success rate on cancer is miserably low. And second, his was the primary voice speaking out consistently to demonstrate that not only did Laetrile therapy obviously provide "some" relief for cancer patients, but it was nontoxic, at least in any meaningful sense. These two realities sharpened his appetite for the coming battles.

He was not alone, of course, in questioning the viral theory of cancer

— the notion that somehow cancer is an alien, outside disease — and that it must therefore be treated with radical means: chemotherapy, radiation, and surgery. If the premise that cancer is an "outside-caused" disease is valid, then the methods of cut it out, burn it out, and cut it off are valid. If, instead, cancer is an intrinsic condition — a metabolic malfunction — then the trinty of chemotherapy, radiation, and surgery constitute the often useless and always dangerous treatment of symptoms, not the treatment or even the determination of causes.

Medical history is replete with examples of such well-intentioned if ill-founded practices. The analogy of syphilis comes to mind. It took medicine hundreds of years to learn that syphilis is a general, pervasive disease of which skin ulceration is only a symptom. Even so, the treatment of symptoms did, from time to time, cause palliation.

Dean Burk, whose doctorate is a Ph.D., not an M.D., was continually distressed to note the toxicity of the most popular "modern" approach to cancer control: chemotherapy. Chemotherapy is the treatment of cancer tissues and/or disease-causing micro-organisms by chemicals that have a specific, poisonous effect on the tissues or micro-organisms. Reduced to simplest terms in cancer therapy, it is the treatment of neoplasms with poisons. All of the chemotherapeutic agents in cancer therapy are poisonous to a greater or lesser degree, and some of them are extremely dangerous. Even in those authentic cases where they retard or arrest cancer tumors, their effect on the body ranges from mildly to highly poisonous. Too, only a few decades ago chemotherapy was thought to be practically as unwarranted as orthodox medicine believes the Laetrile approach is today.

The mildest effects of chemotherapy parallel something on the order of narcotic withdrawal symptoms — cramps, lessened appetite, growing weakness, nausea, and diarrhea. In advanced symptoms, hair frequently falls out and other unpleasant side effects have been noted. One study in the *New York Journal of Medicine* for March 1, 1971, admits a death rate of ten percent — that is, ten percent of the patients die from chemotherapy, not from cancer.

The defense of chemotherapy among oncologists seems almost to be a last-ditch, clutch-at-any-straw affair. In *The Wayward Cell* (University of California Press, 1972), Dr. Victor Richards describes the failure of chemotherapy and, interestingly enough, adds: "Nevertheless, chemotherapy serves an extremely valuable role in keeping patients oriented toward proper medical therapy, and prevents the feeling of being abandoned by the physician in patients with late and hopeless cancers. Judicious employment and screening of potentially useful drugs may also prevent the spread of cancer quackery." Never mind, one might add, the high cost of these toxic drugs in legitimate cancer therapy; even if the patient is harmed, not helped, by chemotherapy, he is better off!

Whenever possible, Burk brought up statements by officialdom and orthodoxy pointing to the low-level five-year survival rates for metastasized (spread) cancer, indicating that in general cancer sufferers can expect only a 7.5 percent five-year survival rate.[2]

Whether or not "objective benefit" from orthodox cancer approaches is that low or not, by 1974 — at least according to National Cancer Institute and California Department of Health spokesmen with whom I spoke — the estimated survival rate seemed better but hardly optimistic. The California department informed me that "the relative five-year survival rate for all cancers (excluding basal and squamous skin cancer and in-situ cancers) is 40 percent." The relative five-year survival rate for patients with early (localized) disease is 68 percent, they added.

In the summer of 1973, Burk quoted ranking researchers to the effect that "85 percent of cancers do not respond to any drugs."[3] Some tumor systems seem virtually unsusceptible of treatment by standard methods; others are susceptible if caught early enough.

Burk did not argue that Laetrile-using physicians were reporting in excess of a 15 percent "objective benefit" in direct cancer therapy (understanding again, that the great majority of patients whom they see are terminal ones), but such therapists do add two major elements: no harmful side effects and much higher percentages of pain relief than the 5 to 15 percent "objective benefit" in patients.

Burk was fond of quoting from the Sixth National Cancer Conference Proceedings in 1968, which was jointly sponsored by the American Cancer Society and the National Cancer Institute. Among the testimony from the conference (and published by Lippincott in 1970) were these statements:

• Robert D. Sullivan, M.D., Department of Cancer Research, Lahey Clinic Foundation, Boston (p. 543): "There has been an enormous undertaking of cancer research to develop anticancer drugs for use in the management of neoplastic diseases in man. However, progress has been slow, and no chemical agents capable of inducing a general curative effect on disseminated forms of cancer have yet been developed."

• James F. Holland, M.D., Roswell Park Memorial Institute, New York State Department of Health, Buffalo, N.Y. (p. 609): "Human cancers are refractory in large part to cure by the chemotherapeutic approaches which have been tried...."

• William Powers, M.D., director, Division of Radiation Therapy, Washington University School of Medicine, St. Louis (p. 33): "Although preoperative and postoperative radiation therapy have been used extensively and for decades, it is still not possible to prove an unequivocal clinical benefit from this combined treatment .... Even if the rate of cure does improve with a combination of radiation and therapy, it is necessary to establish the *cost* in increased morbidity which may occur in patients with or without favorable response to the additional therapy."

• Philip Rubin, M.D., chief, Division of Radiotherapy, University of Rochester Medical School, Strong Memorial Hospital, Rochester, N.Y. (p. 855): "With thousands of lung cancer patients treated by irradiation, the value of radiation therapy should be clearly established or disestablished. The indictment of radiotherapy in the treatment of this disease by Kraut ('The Question of Irradiation Therapy in Lung Cancer,' JAMA 195 (1966): 177-81) is a carefully researched document that has to be considered. The clinical evidence and statistical data in numerous reviews are cited to illustrate that no increase in survival has been achieved by the addition of irradiation."

• Vera Peters, M.D., Princess Margaret Hospital, Toronto, Ont. (p. 163): "Shimkin ('End Results in Cancer of the Breast,' *Cancer* 20 (1967): 1039-43) has shown recently that in carcinoma of the breast, the mortality rate still parallels the incidence rate, thus proving that there has been no true improvement in the successful treatment of the disease over the past thirty years, even though there has been technical improvement in both surgery and radio-therapy during that time."

• Robert L. Egan, M.D., professor of radiology and chief, Mammography Section, Emory University School of Medicine, Atlanta, Ga.; and R. Waldo Powell, M.D., associate professor of surgery, Department of Surgery (p. 153): "The thirty-year monotonous plateau of the death rate for breast cancer has persisted despite physicians' awareness of breast cancer, refinements of methods of inspecting and palpitating the breast, educating women in self-examination, improvements in radiotherapy that include supervoltage, use of more extensive surgical procedures, and the use of chemotherapy and hormones."

• I.E. Gillespie, M.D.; H.T. Debas, M.D.; and F. Kennedy, University Department of Surgery, Western Infirmary, Glasgow, Scotland (p. 421): "Since there is yet no sign that either radio-therapy or chemotherapy can offer real therapeutic benefit to patients with gastric cancer, the main hope at present for either cure, or useful palliation, rests with surgical treatment. The many varied surgical approaches do not seem to have made a great difference to the overall outcome in large series of patients, and it seems unlikely that much improvement can be expected from further developments of surgical technique."

• Saul A. Rosenberg, M.D., associate professor of medicine and radiology, Stanford University School of Medicine, Palo Alto, Calif. (p.

83): "Thus, worthwhile palliation is achieved in many patients; however, there still will be the inevitable relapse of the malignant lymphoma, and, either because of drug resistance or drug intolerance, the disease will recur, requiring modifications of the chemotherapy program and eventually failure to control the disease process. With very few exceptions, cure is not achieved despite the dramatic initial benefit which is seen in so many patients."

• John D. Trelford, M.D., F.R.C.S., Department of Obstetrics and Gynecology, Ohio State University Hospital (p. 379): "At the present time chemotherapy of gynecological tumors does not appear to be have increased life expectancy except in sporadic cases. . . . There appears to be no satisfactory method of determining to which drug a tumor will be sensitive. The only basis of selecting a drug is by past experience. The problem of blind chemotherapy means not only a loss of the effect of the drugs, but also a lowering of the patient's resistance to the cancer cells owing to the toxicity of these agents. . . . At the present time there is no satisfactory method of stimulating or mobilizing the host's immunological defenses to aid in controlling or eradicating the patient's malignancy."

In other words, the most eminent cancer scientists of the day freely acknowledge that the "traditional" methods of treatment — cut, burn, and poison — are not working. But they refuse even to consider such a simple solution as the use of vitamins.

In his lengthy report on Laetrile to Congressman Louis Frey, Jr. on May 30, 1972, Dr. Burk also referred to the May 18, 1972, lecture by Dr. Charles Moertal of the Mayo Clinic at the heavily attended chemotherapy conference held at the National Institute of Health. He quotes Moertal:

> *Perhaps some small and hesitant progress has been made, but it is evident that in this year of 1972 there is no remarkably effective specific therapy for any types of gastro-intestinal carcinoma that cannot be surgically extirpated. There are none that can be accorded the stature of treatment of preference.*
>
> *Our most effective regimens are fraught with risks and side-effects and practical problems, and after this price is paid by all the patients we have treated, only a small fraction are rewarded with a transient period of usually incomplete tumor regressions . . . .*
>
> *Our accepted and traditional curative efforts therefore yield a failure rate of 85 percent. These patients with advanced gastrointestinal cancer present us with one of the most frequent major disease problems encountered in medical practice today . . . . The patient with gastrointestinal cancer is still getting the same old 5-Fu he got 14 years ago.[4]*

In the same letter to Rep. Frey, Burk noted: "That the various administrative agencies claim Laetrile is worthless may be dismissed ... as unscientifically based, together with the fact that few or none of such claimants has ever worked personally with Laetrile and patients, nor have they seriously if at all ever visited hospitals and clinics where Laetrile is used, and their alleged medical basis goes back to the 1953 report of the California Cancer Commission which described no patient ever receiving a *total* dosage of Laetrile as great as is now the current standard *daily* dosage (3 grams per day or more)."

While the expensive, toxic cancer drugs were securing minimal benefits for a small number of cancer patients, medical orthodoxy and governmental orthodoxy were mobilized against Laetrile, a state of affairs that exasperated Burk. In his letter to Frey, Burk wrote:

> *Although ... Laetrile utilization in this country is proceeding ... in spite of FDA prohibitions, it is even more so because of unwarranted FDA procedures, and lack of FDA scientific and medical justification for its stand, extending to probable unconstitutionality, concerning which many thousands of cancer-afflicted persons and their relatives and physicians are rapidly becoming aware.*
>
> *... I have hundreds of letters sent to me enclosing FDA information sheets and pronouncements, in which the senders of these letters point out the extensive falsification, duplicity, deviousness, red herrings and literal lies ... promulgated by the FDA with respect to Laetrile, as well as similarly on the part of a limited number of certain high officials (though scarcely ever rank-and-file members) of the American Medical Association, the American Cancer Society, the U.S. Department of Health, Education and Welfare, and state agencies ... .*
>
> *It is becoming evident that the current generation of cancer sufferers is coming to regard the intransigence and palpable lies of the FDA and the above-indicated related organizations with a marked measure of contempt on the basis of prima facie evidence provided by these organizations themselves as to their integrity and credibility and that something of a Boston Tea Party mode of action is being undertaken by an increasing number of cancer sufferers in this country, who intend to be hoodwinked no longer; in short, an active backlash is developing even at the grass-roots level....*

Part of the "FDA procedures" Burk was so vehement about in his letter to Congressman Frey concerned the apparent sidetracking within the bureaucracy of information and reports for the FDA compiled by Mc-Naughton. A special House Committee looked into these and other matters in 1971 to some extent — Burk providing testimony and 400 pages of documentation — but all to no avail.

What spurred a fresh Burk outburst was the letter to Rep. Robert A. Roe from the FDA legislative services division concerning the "evaluation of Laetrile as an anticancer agent," and written as part of the correspondence begun by one of Roe's constituents. It was because the FDA letter mentioned that "*no* evidence of anti-tumor activity has been found in *any* of the tests" that Burk saw fit to bring to public view the results of animal testing conducted by the NCI in the spring of 1973, and with whose conclusions he disagreed. Burk charged that the NCI "coverup" of positive test results on mice amounted to another Washington scandal of "Watergate" dimensions. Burk reviewed the series of tests and cited these findings:

It is quite clear that at the particular dosage of 12.5 mg Laetrile (amygdalin MF) per kilogram of mouse a statistically highly significant activity of Laetrile against Lewis mouse lung cancer was indeed observed in these NCI-directed studies . . . .

Furthermore, the NCI-observed ILS (increased life span) values of 41, 51, and 30 percent (average 41 percent) with the Lewis lung cancer in 30 mice (three groups of 10 each) given 12.5 mg Laetrile/kg of mouse daily on days 7-15 after tumor inoculation, are not only above the conventionally accepted minimum significance value of 25 percent ILS for mouse cancers in general, but other data on file in the NCI indicate that very few of the common anticancer chemotherapeutic agents show any significant anticancer activity at all against Lewis lung cancer. . . .

You may wonder, Congressman Roe, why anyone should go to such pains and mendacity to avoid conceding what happened in the NCI-directed experiment. Such an admission and concession is crucially central.

Once any of the FDA-NCI-AMA-ACS hierarchy so much as concedes that Laetrile anti-tumor efficacy was indeed even once observed in NCI experimentation, a permanent crack in the bureaucratic armor has taken place that can widen indefinitely by further appropriate experimentation.

For this reason, I rather doubt that experimentation of the type indicated by me in the foregoing paragraph will be continued or initiated. On the contrary, efforts probably will be made, as they already have, to "explain away" the already-observed positive efficacy by vague and unscientific modalities intended to mislead, along early Watergate lines of corruption, including eventually futile arrogance. . . .[5]

On July 10, 1973, or a week following Burk's letter to Congressman Roe, the NCI associate director for drug research and development announced in a letter to Ralph Glaser, president, Citizens National Committee for Better Health, that "in the case of amygdalin MF there has been a considerable amount of publicity regarding the tests that have been carried out . . . in view of that fact, we have decided to proceed with some additional studies." Shortly thereafter came Burk's announcement in Los Angeles that the Memorial Sloan-Kettering Cancer Center had also undertaken independent studies of the substance.

At the end of 1973, Dr. Burk had become verbally enthusiastic about yet another unorthodox approach to cancer, hydrazine sulfate, a chemical both common and inexpensive and whose use in cancer paralleled the Warburg theory with which the biochemist had earlier associated himself. Indeed, he told me early in 1974 that he believed the chemical might be one of cancer's best battlers, along with Laetrile. Unlike vitamin B-17, hydrazine sulfate, whose experimentation was fledgling but swiftly growing, was not touted as a natural preventative of the disease. "In August (1973) twenty to thirty people were taking hydrazine sulfate. By October-November it was 200 to 300. Now it's several thousand," Dr. Burk reported.

Clinical trials were planned for the Memorial Sloan-Kettering Cancer Center, and other tests were under way elsewhere.[6] Early results were inconclusive and animal work is continuing. More than one observer exulted that in Laetrile and hydrazine sulfate might lie the ultimate answer to the prevention and control of the dread disease. Burk was not all that optimistic: "It's quite possible that hydrazine sulfate or a drug like it will alter the course of cancer, much as insulin alters diabetes, so a person might live an essentially normal life with the disease . . . instead of lying in a hospital bed waiting for the end," he told the *National Enquirer*.

Dr. Joseph Gold, of the Syracuse Cancer Research Institute in New York State, originator of the hydrazine-sulfate theory and the early therapies based on it, had been drawn into the study of hydrazine-sulfate — used as a rocket fuel both in Nazi Germany and later in the United States — by the work on cancer-cell metabolism done by Otto Warburg at Berlin's Max Planck Institute. The latter had demonstrated that glycolysis is the major source of energy in cancer cells. It is the action of the cancer tumor in recycling its wastes and converting normal body mass into tumor substrate that causes an enormous energy drain on normal cells. When the body can no longer compensate for the enormous drain of energy caused by the tumor action, weight loss and debilitation quickly occur.

The answer to interrupting this degenerative metabolic process, he decided, was to inhibit gluconeogenesis — the synthesizing of glucose in the liver and kidney cortex. This can be done by blocking a "pivotal" enzymatic reaction in the gluconeogenesis process. Several chemicals will accomplish the blockage but hydrazine sulfate does it the best, he claims.

Dr. Gold's institute reported on September 26, 1973 that the substance had been used in limited numbers of human patients with advanced disease. "Favorable responses in a wide array of different kinds of cancers have been reported with this drug in many of these patients, the principal benefits being prompt cessation of weight loss and regaining of weight, restoration of strength and vigor, marked diminution of pain, restoration of well-being, and cessation of symptoms of the disease," the institute stated. "There have been no reports of serious side effects of sickness, unlike the drugs now used to treat cancer. Hydrazine sulfate was demonstrated by Dr. Gold to be a powerful tumor inhibitor in previously published animal studies," it added. Dr. Gold recited several spectacular cases of virtual restoration to normal-life activities on the part of terminal patients who took hydrazine-sulfate capsules.

Dr. Burk told me it was still too early to make sweeping claims about the substance, but that so far it had been shown to be nontoxic, a factor recommending it, along with Laetrile, in cancer treatment. His enthusiasm for hydrazine sulfate did not achieve the same level as the enthusiasm other metabolic physicians expressed for Laetrile and by 1976 early results with the substance were mixed.

In 1974, Dr. Burk reached the mandatory retirement age of 70 and stepped down from his post. "That doesn't mean I'm going to sit back and stay silent," the peppery biochemist said. No indeed. In 1975-1976 Burk was spearheading an informational campaign warning of the link between cancer and fluoridated water.[7]

Perhaps his answer to a *Los Angeles Times* question on how he has stood up against unyielding bureaucracy so long in his one-man inside battle for the fair testing of Laetrile best sums up his philosophy: "If you will tell the utter, absolute truth, it is remarkable how most of your problems are solved. It simplifies life tremendously. If you start telling half the truth or three-quarters of the truth, they'll get you."

CHAPTER TWELVE

The McNaughton Epoch

IF ONE DIVIDES "Laetrile history" into the period of its pioneering and first rejection by orthodoxy (1920s to 1953) and the advent of Laetrile as a political as well as medical movement (1972 to the present), he will find the first intermittent epoch occupied by the efforts and activities of The McNaughton Foundation, whose founder-president is as key to the whole story as are the Krebses and early developers of its use.

For Andrew R. L. McNaughton, the shadowy — and quite fascinating — adventurer, scientific thinker and iconoclast — projected Laetrile, and Laetrile production, onto an international scale. Because his name was so linked to the product form of vitamin B-17, even when he no longer had any direct commercial interest in the substance, he was referred to by the American press as the "kingpin" of the "international smuggling ring" between Mexico and the United States.

He became a target for *ad-hominem* attacks on Laetrile because of his globe-girdling multiplicity of interests which, when selectively examined and then tied to Laetrile, *could* be inferentially used to discredit the substance.

Is he what orthodoxy has said — a man with Mafia ties? An international adventurer who had been an arms purveyor (or gun-runner) to both Fidel Castro and the founders of modern Israel? He has been all those things — in a sense — and much more. A complicated personality who never gave me any doubt as to his long-term interests in humanitarianism, McNaughton has indelibly left his mark on Laetrile and the entire movement for metabolic therapy.

His Foundation was established in 1956 as a nonprofit research foundation and, despite its known affiliation with Laetrile and its early efforts to research and legalize Laetrile in Canada and the United States, the Foundation — and McNaughton — have been interested in a wide spectrum of ideas on the fringes of science.

"The attention of the McNaughton Foundation is focused upon transforming into reality new solutions to the problems of mankind, not on commercial developments per se or ivory tower research or educational goals," says the organization's statement of "purpose and operation." It was set up, he said, "to look at new ideas, pick the best ones, and help them get going — to finance innovative approaches to medicine and to close the time-lag between inception and implementation." These innovative ideas have included, aside from Laetrile, vitamin therapy and metabolic medicine itself, new approaches to the problems of aging, Dr. Krebs' pangamic aid (vitamin B-15), new therapies for diabetes and heart disease — and, increasingly, aspects of parapsychology and their relationship to overall health. His, and the Foundation's, interest had moved far more into this area by 1976, since by then he believed that total metabolic therapy involving vitamin B-17 and a spectrum of vitamins and minerals provided the *physical* answer to cancer and predicted that "we'll have to spend the next 10 years proving that the mind is even *more* important in therapy."

For years, McNaughton was anywhere where the Laetrile action in research and development was underway — in Mexico, Monte Carlo, Spain or West Germany, where there are or have been Laetrile-producing facilities, or at the Krebs family mansion in San Francisco. Much of the time, The Foundation has literally operated out of his hip pocket and from post office boxes in Sausalito and San Ysidro, California, the latter, perhaps puckishly, labelled Box B-17.

A self-sustaining business and engineering consultant, the graying but vigorous scion of one of Canada's most distinguished families (though he was actually born in England) is the son of General A. G. L. McNaughton, the commander of the Canadian Armed Forces in World War II. The elder McNaughton was also a president of the United Nations Security Council. "My father was president of the National Research Council in Canada. I was brought up in a scientific atmosphere," he recalls.

His education included a four-year classical course under the Jesuits at Loyola College, Montreal; electrical engineering at the Royal Military College, Kingston, Ontario; geology and mining studies at McGill University, Montreal; and business administration at Alexander Hamilton Institute. He served as a pilot in the Royal Canadian Air Force from 1939 to 1946, winning the Air Force Cross for his performance as a test pilot. Indeed, he was the RCAF's chief test pilot and commanded the air arm's Experimental Test and Development Centre. His scientific memberships span the spectrum from the Royal Society of Medicine and the New York Academy of Sciences to the Point Reyes (California) Bird Observatory.

McNaughton does not hesitate to discuss his other intriguing credentials — arms purveyor to Cuba and Israel, for which he was both made an "honorary citizen of Cuba" and officially thanked by Israeli officials for his Middle Eastern efforts. His exploits as a double agent (arms supplier for the Batista government while diverting the same to Castro as an under-cover member of the July 16 Movement) assumed at times Hollywood-esque proportions.

While many have sought to disparage McNaughton's "politics," the British-born innovator tried to set the record straight when he wrote (for the *Montreal Star*) his memoirs as a double agent and as a supporter of Castro Cuba's first non-Communist president, Dr. Manuel Urrutia: "I believe it is the duty of us all to stand up to dictatorships. It is our duty, but it is not an opportunity that is given to every man. When it is given, as it was to me, what ought a man to do? Mind his business (or) do what he can so that one segment of humanity can taste freedom? I chose the latter course and this would always be my choice."

It was not, however, the Cuban interlude which was more frequent-ly used to tar McNaughton, and therefore Laetrile, but his alleged "Ma-fia connections." And what were they?

When the McNaughton Foundation was operating quite legally in Canada, the sister of an alleged Mafia figure was "kept alive for many years," McNaughton claims. It is because her brother was "very grateful" and asked what he could do that three gifts (of $100,000, $20,000 and $10,000) were made available through a third party to the Foundation. "So that was my Mafia involvement," McNaughton told me.

In 1973, the *Financial Post* in Canada in a lengthy article attempted to link McNaughton and the company he had once set up (International Biozymes Ltd., later Biozymes International Ltd.), with one Joseph (Bayonne Joe) Zicarelli, imprisoned in 1971 at Trenton State Prison, New Jersey, on a 10-to-15-year gambling conspiracy charge. Zicarelli, identified as a "major mob figure," was also described as a principal Biozymes share-holder.

McNaughton had set up Biozymes in 1961 as a profit-making corporation and continued to make Laetrile until the Canadian Depart-ment of National Health and Welfare banned its distribution. The com-pany was specifically set up, he recalled, because a non-profit, tax-exempt organization such as the McNaughton Foundation could not, under Cana-dian law, be sued for recovery of damages and no Canadian pharma-ceutical company would produce Laetrile for test purposes unless they could recover possible losses, except for Delmar Chemicals, Ltd. Biozymes served the purpose of being a profit-making company, but in 1963, when the Canadian clampdown against Laetrile occurred, McNaughton got rid of "all my shares" in Biozymes and it was taken over by others, he said.

The *Financial Post* article, however, helped to create the ongoing illu-sion of Mafia and mobsters in the McNaughton — and thus the Laetrile — camp. By dwelling on the Mafia, Biozymes and Bayonne Joe, and also a case of stock manipulation (due particularly to a complicated case in Canada, whose established powers never forgave him for championing Laetrile), enough imagery was produced to attempt to discredit Mc-Naughton. Then, add Ernst T. Krebs Jr.'s lack of "earned" degrees, and mix liberally with John Birch Society members militating in the fast-growing Committee for Freedom of Choice in Cancer Therapy, Inc., and professional propagandists could have a field day besmirching Laetrile.

Added to the imagery were the realities that product-form Laetrile in the United States was available solely on the "black market" and that some people involved in its use made profits from it. The cost of Laetrile both in the United States and at the Contreras Clinic in Mexico, which McNaughton had helped set up, was used as a kind of propaganda club by anti-Laetrile forces, a "now-they're-soaking-the-desperate" variety of propaganda. In the November 1973 issue of *Today's Health*, for instance, a severe attack on Doctors Krebs and Contreras was levelled, suggesting Laetrile was a big business bilking desperate terminal cancer patients.[1] The claim was made that the true price of manufacture from raw material was no more than two cents per tablet — which, as Dr. Stewart Jones pointed out in a rebuttal letter, was about as honest as saying that the true cost of radiation therapy should be 2 cents per treatment since "the raw material, electricity, costs about 10 cents per kilowatt."

Despite "establishment" efforts to continue casting McNaughton in the role of chief Laetrile smuggler and worldwide amygdalin gray-eminence, by the time this was written his Foundation's sole financial interest was in the patent it held on the freeze-drying (lyophilization) process — now irrelevant since lyophilization is no longer part of the process. Indeed, facing smuggling charges in the 1976 blanket indictments against the "international Laetrile smuggling ring," McNaughton declared his liabilities exceeded his assets and was represented by a court-appointed attorney.

Although some American-made Laetrile was circulating in the U.S. by 1976, most of the material (and all the injectable Laetrile) was coming from the Mexican laboratories (most of whose raw materials came from California) and some from European sources. "These factories won't supply the American market after Laetrile becomes 'legal' in the U.S.," McNaughton told me. "We give free courses on how to manufacture the stuff to anyone who will listen. We have no secrets. The factories all use apricot kernels but some are also experimenting with bitter almonds, peaches, prunes, cherries, Johnson grass and sorghum. Four organizations are researching the production of synthetic materials."

Claiming he had "absolutely no financial interest in Laetrile," Mc-Naughton was a most unlikely international kingpin for "international smuggling" when this was written. He also insisted he was anxiously awaiting the day for established orthodoxy to sanction Laetrile officially so he could feel totally free to move into his next major area of interest, which is the role of the mind in cancer in particular and in health in general.

By 1976, the Foundation was mostly a two-man affair — McNaughton as President, and Stephen Zalac, a specialist in nutrition, as vice president. It maintained an extensive and impressive international advisory board, including such names as former American Association for the Advancement of Science President Chauncey D. Leake, and Laetrile pioneers Gurchot, Krebs and Navarro, and professors in the Soviet Union.[2]

McNaughton was by then insisting that "within a short time Laetrile and its ancillary therapy will be the established way of treating cancer — and then science may have to convince the establishment that the mind is greater in importance."

By no means, of course, do Krebs and many other pragmatic scientists share McNaughton's lifelong enthusiasm over things parapsychological, but several do, including some of the multi-degreed savants who are Foundation advisors.

I had not been aware of this interest of McNaughton's during the time I interviewed the first series of hard-core terminal cases referred to earlier. In those cases, as noted, attitude and religious faith seemed to be playing some kind of role.

In the meantime, Jean Shinoda Bolen, M.D., had published in her husband's magazine, *Psychic* (which I had helped, in a small way, to bring into existence), some of the results of the work of Major O. Carl Simonton, then chief of radiation therapy at Travis Air Force Base, California. She wrote (in "Meditation and Psychotherapy in the Treatment of Cancer"): ". . . Simonton is thoroughly convinced that one's state of mind has to do with the development of cancer and must be reckoned with in treating it as well. 'The mind, the emotions, and the attitude of a patient,' he steadfastly maintains, 'play a role in both the development of a disease, cancer included, and the response that a patient has to any form of treatment.' "

In a two-year study of 152 cancer patients he treated, Dr. Simonton stated that their improved or unimproved conditions correlated to their degree of participation in his special treatment program and their positive or negative attitudes.

Dr. Simonton had begun his interest in the new approach to cancer in 1969 at the University of Oregon Medical Center, when he noted that certain patients "inexplicably" lived longer or were "unexpectedly" cured during radiation therapy — patients who beat enormous odds in advanced, terminal cancer. In talking with these patients, he detected a consistent, positive, even stubborn attitude of "I can't die until such and such happens." Then there were the patients who said they wanted to live but whose actions said otherwise — persons with lung cancer who continued to smoke, those with liver cancer who continued to drink — and those who frequently said things like "Maybe I deserved this" or "It's probably punishment for what I did."

Further, Dr. Simonton heard patients describe their life situation at the time their cancers arose — phrases such as "I felt trapped" or "I hadn't much to live for" were frequent. Somehow, the mind had determined the need for death, and the body had responded, finding a way — cancer. Sensing that the mind might very well have a role in inducing cancer, Dr. Simonton turned his attention to whether it could not therefore also have a role in inhibiting the disease. He came up with a series of meditative techniques involving relaxation and visualization and also educating victims about their cancers.

In the survey of 152 patients treated with his visualization method, 20 showed responses Dr. Simonton described as "excellent." Of these, all were said to be highly motivated to live and cooperated well. Of those with no relief of symptoms or only mild relief, none had been fully cooperative or positively motivated. Except for two cases — patients who showed good results despite negative attitudes — all results showed improvement or unimprovement in correlation to their attitudes and degrees of participation.

None of this is mysterious to McNaughton. Cancer has become, he says, "a socially acceptable way to commit suicide."

At the end of 1973, The McNaughton Foundation published *Physicians' Handbook of Vitamin B-17 Therapy*, which combined the established Laetrile therapy with "the role of positive thinking." The booklet carried this preface by Andrew McNaughton:

> *Cancer, like many diseases, is an expression of conflict between the living organism and hostile factors in the total environment. The mind, through the nervous system, can influence this conflict constructively or destructively. Hence to a varying degree cancer is something which the mind is permitting to happen to the body. From contact with more than 5,000 cancer patients over the past 15 years it is apparent that for many of them cancer was a form of socially acceptable suicide. For best results under vitamin B-17 therapy the patient must cooperate mentally and physically, positively and actively, in his treatment.*
>
> *More often than not, Quitters die, Fighters live.*

CHAPTER THIRTEEN

The Committee:
Leading the Way to a New Era

BY 1976, an American Cancer Society official was in a sense correct in labelling "Laetrile the number-one problem in cancer quackery — and the Committee for Freedom of Choice in Cancer Therapy, Inc., the number-one problem in Laetrile."

The remark was testimony to the fact that the California-based Committee had, in four years, become the major advocacy organization for the legalization of Laetrile, as well as the key voice battling for freedom of choice in medicine and the vindication of metabolic therapy.

Organized in virtually every state of the union, Committee efforts had secured the first "freedom of choice" act in Alaska and were vigorously pushing for legalization in many other states. The Committee-sponsored doctors' workshops, held across the country, were educating inquiring physicians on cancer and metabolic therapy in which vitamin B-17 plays the central role.

Symposia in cities large and small, showings of filmstrips in schools, churches and union halls, letter-writing campaigns, media interviews, cultivation of elected officials all played roles in the Committee's multi-faceted approach to the Laetrile problem.

It was without a doubt the explosive, rapid growth of the Committee after the arrest of California physician John A. Richardson in 1972 which brought the turnaround in the Laetrile story and moved the fight for Laetrile into a whole new political dimension: the fight for freedom itself.

When federal smuggling indictments were issued against Committee President Robert W. Bradford, first, and later against Vice President J. Franklin Salaman (and naming Committee Executive Director Beverly Newkirk as an "unindicted co-conspirator"), they represented "establishment" efforts to smash the growing ad hoc movement once and for all.

But establishment forces learned they were not dealing with criminals and smugglers, but with men and women who were — incredibly enough — essentially involved in the vitamin B-17 movement first and foremost out of humanitarian concerns.

This reality was the hardest one for much of the media and the powers that be to swallow. Attempts were made to dismiss the Committee itself as a smuggling racket, its leaders as criminals enriching themselves. If that illusion could not stick, then the Committee, due to the marked presence of John Birch Society members in its ranks, was denounced as a front group for the JBS.

The efforts to smear the Committee and its leaders were not all venal; some of them came from the extreme difficulty 20th-century America has in accepting the fact that people might be involved in something which has the aura of illegality because they are motivated by humane concerns.

As a Committee founder and indicted alleged smuggler Salaman put it: "Does it make sense that a smuggler who is supposed to be making millions of dollars off of what he is smuggling would spend five years of his life trying to legalize it?"

An independent businessman and successful entrepreneur, Salaman is the scion of a wealthy and highly respected California family. A graduate of Northwestern University with a master's in business and a former champion debater in college, Salaman was, at the age of nineteen, the youngest captain in the U.S. Navy; wounded in the Pacific theater, he spent a year in a hospital before his discharge. An occasional politician, Salaman was well off long before he knew anything about Laetrile. Yet regional media delighted in pointing to the opulent Salaman family mansion, the Salaman family vehicles, and the fact the Salamans had a Lake Tahoe lodge and yacht as evidence that somehow the San Francisco Peninsula family was reaping huge dividends from Laetrile. To the contrary, he has been one of the major contributors to the movement.

The fact is, the fiftyish businessman did *not* need Laetrile to enhance either his lifestyle or interfere with his acquaintances.

Salaman was already a nationally known speaker on American liberties and government encroachment before a mutual friend, Dr. Richardson, was arrested on cancer quackery charges, and before his wife, Maureen, caring for a terminal cancer patient, knew anything about Laetrile.

But when the traumatic moment of the Richardson arrest occurred, the Salamans — husband and wife — could no more have stayed out of the fight than they could have watched a man dying of thirst and not provide water. I say this from personally knowing these people, leaders of a national movement who simply are not the confidence agents, profiteers and criminals the established forces made them out to be.

Salaman's long-time friend, Robert W. Bradford, hardly needed Laetrile for enrichment purposes, either.

A scientist trained in physics and electronics engineering, and already backgrounded in medicine and science because he comes from a medical family, Bradford gave up a career position at Stanford University, where he worked on the Stanford Linear Accelerator, and also abandoned his electronics products ownership to throw himself completely into the Laetrile cause.

Across the country and at the outset of Committee efforts, Bradford and Salaman as individuals — *not* as Committee officers — boldly announced that they would see to it that doctors who needed Laetrile in the United States would get it, and that they would help patients who wished to be in the care of such physicians to get the two sides together.

"There was a period when Laetrile supplies were being choked off from doctors who wanted to get it and couldn't," Bradford recalls. "Let's face it: people were dying. There was an utter need for supplies of quality-controlled Laetrile to reach physicians. Frank and I tried to help fill that need."

Bradford and Salaman did not hide their intentions or goals — they openly announced them in public meetings. They insisted throughout that they were not smugglers, and demanded of the authorities that they be told once and for all if receiving supplies of Laetrile constituted a crime. After several years of seeing to it that physicians received Laetrile, after openly announcing and implementing their intentions, the pair received their answer from the U.S. government with the "conspiracy to smuggle" indictments and the attempt to link them with an "international ring."

From the beginning, the Bradford-Salaman collaboration was not based on the desire for smuggling profits, but to fight for legal, open distribution of this *natural food substance* for medical use, and to champion the rapidly growing cause of metabolic therapy or holistic medicine. Indeed, their securing of attorneys under Committee sponsorship established, in the Richardson and Privitera cases, the validity and legality of B-17 use in metabolic therapy despite state laws against Laetrile, as we have seen. More important, such efforts brought to the fore the nature of the opposition not only to Laetrile, but to the whole concept of natural therapy and prevention, and it is this fact which explains the degree of the venom directed against the rapidly growing Committee and its leadership.

Also from the beginning, the Committee founders sought to impose stringent quality control on Laetrile, both in injectable and tablet form, to insure quality just as their activities, they hoped, could guarantee quantity. A key function of the Committee as late as 1976 was to monitor the various Laetriles being distributed in the United States to make certain they were "quality" products.

171

The Committee also sought to rebut the charges that the cost of Laetrile represented a monumental "ripoff" of desperate cancer patients, and was instrumental in attempting to set price lids for the substance on what the "establishment" regarded as a black market.

In 1974, an agreement was worked out with the Mexican government on maximum wholesale and retail prices in Mexico, a binding accord inasmuch as the Mexican government officially sets drug prices. The effort was to alert U.S. consumers to the true costs of the substance. The agreed prices then were a maximum retail price of $9 per three-gram vial and a maximum retail price on a 500-milligram tablet of $1 — figures for products coming from the CytoPharma de Mexico laboratory in Tijuana, the primary purveyor of Laetrile in North America.

By 1976, the American (or "black market") Laetrile was selling at $10 or $11 per vial and tablets anywhere from 90 cents to a dollar — these were the *real* figures, in distinction to the "up to $50" figure claimed by state and federal governments in their crackdown on Laetrile distribution and their efforts to tar Laetrile distributors as profit-motivated hyenas salivating after the carrion of the desperate.

Although scattered abuses of the cost of Laetrile had indeed occurred, *all* such abuses, based on black-marketeering and smuggling, were attributable more than anything else to the U.S. government and the medical establishment, which had turned Laetrile into a sinister substance on the order of 1920s bootleg whiskey. Moreover, the "black market" markup of about *10 percent* hardly left much room for massive profiteering — and the cost of the product Laetrile over the cost of raw materials from which it is made remained far under the cost of "orthodox" drugs as contrasted with the costs of raw materials from which they are produced.

The hullabaloo over Laetrile use raised by the establishment in 1976, and repeated faithfully in the "establishment" press, including the *New York Times* News Service and major press syndicates, claimed that visitors to the Tijuana clinics, where treatment was quite legal, were being "ripped off " — and that Laetrile patients receiving Laetrile-based therapy in the United States were equally being stripped of their last few dollars for a quack cancer cure. This was the criminal-aura background against which the public activities of the Committee operated, the image against which Committee leaders had to struggle.

Press reports referred to millions of dollars of profits off quackery accruing to Dr. Contreras and the Del Rio brothers in Mexico, and to Dr. Richardson and the Laetrile-using physicians north of the border. They sought to link such alleged profits with the Committee and even to Andrew McNaughton, who by the time of the federal indictments had long since abandoned direct interest in Laetrile production and the Laetrile clinics in Mexico.

Where was the "ripoff"? By Dr. Richardson in California, who had a staff of 22 and operated an expanding clinic and who had been using amygdalin for years? By Dr. Contreras, who had been operating an expanding clinic since 1963? These were the alleged "millionaires" with profits estimated on gross earnings and based on anecdotal "evidence." Articles referring to such sums never, of course, questioned how many millions of dollars "orthodox" cancer specialists and surgeons were salting away in the U.S. or how many millions were being made annually by prestigious medical institutions whose cut-burn-poison approach to cancer was sending far more people to their graves than were being rescued.

As to costs in Tijuana: the normal expense for treatment at the major clinics by 1976 (Dr. Contreras' Del Mar Medical Center and the Del Rio brothers' Cydel Clinic) varied between $900 to $2,000 for an average three-week stay, a figure usually including all board and lodging and frequently including a six-months supply of medicine sent home with the patient. This writer interviewed patient after patient from both clinics, none of whom had felt "ripped off" and many of whom were in excellent condition to compare the costs of their treatment at home and the same costs in Tijuana.

The *Rochester* (Minnesota) *Post-Bulletin*, whose January 1974 series on Laetrile was one of the few *objective*, in-depth reporting jobs done on the controversial treatment, found the Tijuana costs quite reasonable: A $10 first-office call, $7 for subsequent office visits, a $3 clinical service fee per visit, and a $30 daily charge for private hospital rooms, a figure increased slightly by 1976.

The June 1976 issue of *The Choice*, the Committee's official publication, carried testimony from patients who had been treated both in the U.S. and in Mexico. One patient, reporting complete recovery from cancer after three months in Tijuana, claimed his total treatment cost had been $11 a day — and that the examination he underwent in a Texas hospital simply to verify his claims of total cancer control had cost him $800, along with $50 per-visit interviews with his American doctors. A 21-year-old coed who reported in the same publication on her dramatic total-recovery case said it had cost her $2,500 for treatment entirely within the U.S.

It is common for a terminal, metastasized cancer patient when treated in the U.S.A. to spend a *total* of between $30,000 and $50,000 — quite aside from the American Cancer Society's perhaps relevant statistic that a "typical hospital stay" for a cancer patient averages 16 days and $1,500. What the ACS doesn't point out is that there are usually *many* hospital stays, and expensive continuing medication and treatment. The *total* care cost of cancer patients in the United States, as contrasted with those who made the "Tijuana connection," is monstrous. It includes hospital rooms of $100 or more per day, expensive anesthesiology, prohibitively expensive surgery, costly radiation, expensive — and dangerous — chemotherapy, and expensive doctors' calls, followup visits, admission fees, insurance premiums and tests of all kinds. The only *real* "ripoff" in cancer, indeed, tends to be that practiced by orthodox medicine in the U.S.

To bring this total picture to the public became a major part of Committee propaganda and advertising efforts, and for this purpose, in no small part, the Committee converted what began as a small, mimeographed newsletter into a national publication — *The Choice*.

Maureen Salaman, the attractive and dynamic wife of Vice President Frank Salaman, became associate editor of the publication and remains one of the most outspoken champions of freedom of choice. Deeply committed to revealing the truth about Laetrile, Maureen became a one-woman crusader, contacting newsrooms, television stations, and news service bureaus with information, and offering a rapid-fire verbal presentation of the meaning of freedom of choice for all who would listen.

It had been through caring for her friend Helen Sweet in the last six cancer-wracked months of her life that brought her to Laetrile and vitamin therapy, Maureen recalled, but even before that she had campaigned for conservatism, Christian fundamentalism and the reduction of government encroachment in the lives of citizens.

In both written and verbal presentations laced with Biblical quotations and exhortations, Maureen Salaman took on the established forces and dared them to do battle, and even with a tone of forgiveness. "I am enormously enjoying forgiving (Deputy U.S. Attorney) Herb Hoffman and the *New York Times* and its hundreds of imitators for taking this noblest of battles to preserve our freedoms and save lives and through lies and innuendoes make it look like a cheap charade performed for money," she wrote in *The Choice*.

Committee chairmen in some areas became involved in the distribution not only of information — books, pamphlets, film cassettes — but also of apricot and peach kernels, the highly nitrilosidic natural foods which authorities began attempting to remove from the shelves of health food stores. Despite their insistence that Congress had passed no law against apricot and peach kernels, and the reality that possession of natural seeds is no crime, distributors of this natural material continued to be "leaned on," through 1975 and 1976, either not to sell their merchandise or to make it a back-room enterprise.

And some Chairmen fell into the toils of the law through actual malicious prosecution. Steve Harrison, a Greensboro, N.C., pharmacist and Committee chairman, was sent to federal prison in summer 1976 because he had sold three pieces from his private gun collection — without a license — to two undercover state agents who had worked into his confidence and represented themselves as gun collectors.

While Harrison admitted he should not have made the sales, he was considerably irked that the agents had spent so much time in literally cajoling and baiting him until he made the sales more out of a frustrated desire to be rid of the nuisances than make money. But few doubted that Harrison was essentially a target for prosecutory wrath because of his open advocacy of Laetrile (his business cards read "Laetrile Works — You Bet Your Life") and freedom of choice. State and federal agents even raided his pharmacy after they had earlier visited him for a "routine inspection." During the raid they confiscated peach kernels, books and magazine articles dealing with Laetrile, and a supply of the latter Harrison — who swore he had never made a dime off vitamin B-17 — was holding for a patient.

The prosecution of Harrison in North Carolina paralleled the State of California harassment against Dr. Stewart Jones, already exonerated by the state medical board of all but one Laetrile-connected charge, and a conservative San Francisco Peninsula book store owner, Douglas Hoiles. Both were arrested for alleged involvement in providing Laetrile as a "cure for cancer." But in sworn testimony for their defense attorney, an undercover state agent revealed she had been pressured to lie about what Jones and Hoiles said, and also coerced to sign this false statement about their arrests.

Because of such prosecutions, which only reinforced the Committee position that the central issue in the Laetrile controversy was politics rather than science, the organization redoubled its lobbying efforts.

As this is written, the Committee for Freedom of Choice in Cancer Therapy, Inc., is the acknowledged leader in the crusade for legal Laetrile and for the recognition and legalization of metabolic therapy, which it clearly perceives as the wave of the medical future.

It has opened a whole new era in the medical revolution and has established a tax-deductible foundation, the Cancer Prevention and Research Foundation, to help carry on this revolution through research in the holistic approach to metabolic diseases.

What had begun in a private meeting of a half-dozen people in California rallying around an embattled doctor had grown into a national political movement.

Bradford, the courageous President of the committee, never lost sight of what was really at stake.

As he told *The Review of the News* in September 1976:

"The issues here are clear. Physicians and patients either have freedom of choice or they do not. If they do not, then who gave the government the right to take it away from them? And if this right is lost in medicine, where will it be lost next?"

CHAPTER FOURTEEN

Treating Cancer
With a Food Factor

THE LAETRILE THERAPY, as derived from the work of the Krebses, the research of scientists in several parts of the world, and the practical experiences of doctors such as John Richardson and Lawrence McDonald in the United States and Ernesto Contreras in Mexico, is based on the idea that cancer is a metabolic disease and that a combination of intrinsic and extrinsic factors will retard it once it is present. The corollary to this, of course, is that the same combination of intrinsic and extrinsic factors will probably prevent it from starting!

By 1976, the belief that cancer can be *prevented* simply by increasing the amount of natural vitamin B-17 in the diet became virtually as important a part of the "Laetrile movement" as did the controversy over processed vitamin B-17 (Laetrile) in the management and treatment of the disease.

Established political and scientific forces attempted to construe the Laetrile metabolic therapy as a gimmicky way to skirt the Laetrile "ban" and California state laws. But vitamin B-17 as part of a total nutritional therapy was indeed coming into its own; it was finding champions in such metabolic physicians as Oregon's Dr. E. Paul Wedel and interest among such pioneers of preventive medicine as Dr. Harold Harper of California, head of the American Academy of Medical Preventics (AAMP), which was blazing new trails in what was becoming known as "holistic" medicine, or whole treatment for the whole man instead of "fragmented" medicine for the treatment of crises.

The argument which swirled around two of the three trials of Dr. John Richardson (and, later, of Dr. James Privitera) and of the medical board hearing of Dr. Stewart Jones was that the physicians were not treating cancer, at least cancer as traditionally defined, *per se.* The three physicians argued that they were treating the whole person with metabolic therapy, including megavitamins, in which vitamin B-17 played a central role. In effect, they said, they were shoring up the metabolic processes of the whole person so that these processes would do their own "curing" of the disease — which frequently occurs concurrently with other in-salubrious conditions and mineral imbalances.

The laetrilists argue that "lump and bump" manifestations of cancer are symptoms, not root causes, of cancer. Indeed, it is the body's reaction to the explosive trophoblast (cancer) cells that causes the lumps and bumps in the first place. The treatment of such lumps and bumps (most radically, through surgery) is only the treatment of a symptom. An analogy can be made to the treatment of the lesions of syphilis before it was discovered that syphilis had a specific (and in this case extrinsic) cause.

Late in 1973, the McNaughton Foundation issued its *Physician's Handbook of Vitamin B-17 Therapy*. Not mentioning Laetrile by name at all, the booklet stated:

> In vitamin B-17 therapy the cyanide is liberated under safe conditions. Thus adequate dosage is possible without the occurrence of toxic effects. Detoxification occurs in normal mammalian tissue through the action of the enzyme rhodanese in the presence of sulfur-bearing compounds, converting free cyanide to thiocyanate. Cancer cell deficiency of rhodanese may be a determining factor in the effect of the cyanide upon neoplasms.
>
> Hydrolysis of amygdalin (vitamin B-17) releases hydrocyanic acid, benzaldehyde and two sugar molecules.[1]

Pharmacologist Charles Gurchot, Dr. Ernst T. Krebs, Jr.'s mentor, has appended "suggested mechanisms of action" of the vitamin therapy in the booklet this way: Oral doses of vitamin B-17 pass into the intestine where the substance is acted upon by bacterial enzymes. The enzyme complex emulsin breaks amygdalin into four components: hydrocyanic acid, benzaldehyde, prunasin, and mandelonitrile; these components in turn are absorbed into the lymph and portal systems. Cyanide is converted into thiocyanate "probably in the blood circulation, and certainly in the liver by the enzyme of rhodanese in the presence of sulfur-bearing compounds. . . . In cancer patients some thiocyanate finds its way to the site of the cancer lesion."[2]

Prunasin may circulate in the body and reach the malignancy, there hydrolyzing to liberate hydrocyanic acid, benzaldehyde, and a molecule of glucose. Prunasin may also be changed in the liver to mandelonitrile glucuronoside, either by combining with glucuronic acid or by oxidation of the terminal alcohol group of the prunasin glucose molecule. The mandelonitrile absorbed from the intestine goes directly to the liver, where it is converted to glucuronic acid. It may then be excreted as glucuronide or find its way to a malignant lesion.

Dr. Gurchot states that glucosidic enzymes at the lesion may hydrolyze prunasin into its components cyanide, benzaldehyde, and a glucose molecule, and in the process pure mandelonitrile may be released. Mandelonitrile may then undergo spontaneous hydrolysis to hydrocyanic acid and benzaldehyde.

One suggestion emanating out of the Sloan-Kettering tests in 1973 was that mandelonitrile might actually be the primary tool in tumor retardation, rather than cyanide. Barbara J. Culliton, writing in the respected journal *Science* for December 1973 and reporting on the Laetrile tests at S-K, noted:

> *Basically, the idea that has been put forward for years to explain Laetrile's alleged ability to kill cancer cells is that it releases lethal doses of cyanide when it is taken up by a tumor.*
>
> *"Certainly there is some old literature showing that cyanide has anticancer activity," [Dr. Lloyd J.] Old notes. "The question is whether this is so and, if it is, how you can harness the enormous toxicity of cyanide."*
>
> *The question has yet to be answered fully, but there are now some data to suggest that, rather than cyanide, another chemical — mandelonitrile — may be at work.*
>
> *One of the scientists on Old's team looked at Laetrile in human tissues and found that they appear to be "incapable of generating cyanide from amygdalin. It was therefore suggested that mandelonitrile might indeed be the putative therapeutic agent resulting from amygdalin," according to a confidential working report. The possibility is being investigated.*
>
> *Mandelonitrile is at least as toxic as cyanide, Sloan-Kettering researchers point out. The idea behind their work is fairly simple. It may be that there is an enzyme peculiar to tumor cells which is capable of cleaving mandelonitrile from amygdalin, thereby selectively releasing a lethal molecule from one that is nontoxic. As far as is known, amygdalin is relatively safe, even in large doses.[3]*

I found the last remark of particular interest in view of the FDA crackdown on the vitamin B-17-containing food products and the veiled suggestions made by medical orthodoxy that Laetrile is dangerous because of its cyanide content.

Again, as we have seen, even the most ardent laetrilists do not feel they have learned everything about how Laetrile actually "works," and several theories on its mechanism of action have been advanced. The role of Laetrile, and of cyanates themselves, in cancer remains to be far more fully explored.

In his introduction to *Physician's Handbook of Vitamin B-17 Therapy*, Dr. Krebs notes: "Cancer is a chronic metabolic disease in which the host

FREEDOM FROM CANCER

resistance is diminished. All metabolic diseases now prevented or cured
are, without exception, prevented or cured by vitamins, minerals, and
other factors normal to the diet and to the animal economy. By contrast,
no chronic or metabolic disease — or any other disease — *of the host* has
ever been prevented or cured by toxic chemicals or by radiation or by anything else foreign to the natural experience of the organism."

He explains the "totality of the pancreatic enzymes" as the "intrinsic,
surveillant, antineoplastic factor" which, alone, blocks the development of
cancer. Second to them as the intrinsic factor, he says, is the immunological system, particularly in its lymphocytic function. Whatever
can break away the protective "shield" around the cancer (or trophoblast)
cell allows the immunological system to go to work and also to expose it
"to further digestion by the 'deshielding' enzymes themselves."

The control of cancer — called by Krebs "the trophoblast external to
gestation" — is thus not only under the "surveillance" of the intrinsic enzymes and the immunological resources of the host, but it is also, in his
opinion, under the "naturally selected surveillance of dietary or extrinsic
enzymes brought into the organism."

This forms the rationale for the Laetrile therapy's heavy reliance on
fresh and raw plant material rather than on cooked foods, even when the
latter are supplemented with all the known vitamins and required
minerals. "Dietary deprivation of enzymes or vitamins or minerals may be
decisive in the proper functioning of the immunological forces of the
body," Krebs notes in the introduction.

Current Laetrile treatment uses a dosage of three grams of Laetrile
per day, with a range of one to twelve grams per day, the handbook's
"general clinical routine" points out. The upper limits of dosage use are
calculated on the basis of 300 milligrams of vitamin B-17 per kilogram
(2.2 lbs.) of body weight. Hence, the upper limit of dosage for a 154-
pound adult would be about twenty-one grams a day.

By 1975 and 1976, some Laetrile physicians were giving as many as
twelve, and in a few cases, more than twenty, grams per day with no
demonstrable side effects. Based on a number of medical conferences
bringing together the experience of metabolic physicians, the Committee
for Freedom of Choice in Cancer Therapy, Inc., in 1976 elaborated a composite program of clinical applications of vitamin B-17 in which the
starting minimum intravenous dosage is 6 grams or 20 cc daily, increasing
to 9 grams daily for two weeks, with dosages and intravenous use decreasing thereafter as the patient transfers to maintenance use of tablets and
diet.

The substance may be given orally (in tablets ranging from 100-to-
500-milligram doses or broken up and added to soft food), intravenously,

intramuscularly, intrapleurally, intrauterinely, and through direct application. Dosage changes may be determined by the sense of well-being a patient exhibits.

The McNaughton booklet describes a total dosage "in excess of 300 grams" over a period of time as the average amount "in controlling a moderate cancer crisis." A "severe cancer crisis brought under control may be maintained in a quiescent state by the oral administration of 1 gram . . . daily," it adds.

In a general letter to physicians circulated by the Committee for Freedom of Choice in Cancer Therapy, Dr. John A. Richardson, the embattled California physician, stated: "We generally say that a patient who has clinical cancer will be regulated or controlled with 50 grams of Laetrile. That is about 17-20 injections of 3 grams each."

As Laetrile is provided, cancer patients are asked to adhere to a special diet low in or completely avoiding animal proteins and high in fruits and vegetables, preferably raw and whole. Such patients are routinely prescribed pancreatic enzymes, the thinking here being that the ingestion of large amounts of protein has deflected the use of pancreatic enzymes, which digest protein, away from their trophoblast-attacking role, and the intake of a low-animal protein diet *plus* pancreatic enzymes will allow much more natural defense against trophoblast. Bromelain, calcium supplements, and calcium di-orotate are also suggested. Increasingly, metabolic physicians are also prescribing vitamins A, C and E and pangamic acid (vitamin B-15, the other Krebs discovery).

The special dietary regimen, about which there remains certain controversy but which is markedly similar to the "prudent" diet suggested for heart disease prevention and more in alignment with the diets of "primitive" people who suffer little degenerative disease, is recommended for strict adherence for the first several months of therapy but may be gradually relaxed following improvement. Most Laetrile physicians urge their cancer patients to stay on the diet, at least generally, for years.

Based almost solely on fresh fruits and vegetables and/or their fresh juices, and the exclusion of meat (other than the occasional use of fresh fish or poultry cooked without the addition of fat or salt and not treated with hormones), the Laetrile diet is:

Plant Foods: All edible plants and fruits, preferably eaten raw and as fresh as possible. Some may need cooking just enough to make them edible. "Brief and judicious cooking for such periods and at low heat (as done in Chinese restaurants) will not appreciably destroy enzymes in foods." The plant food should be free of additives and preservatives. Whole grains are preferred to refined flour. All sprouted grains are most desirable.

Animal Foods: Fish and poultry should be baked, boiled, or broiled, but never fried, and should be prepared without salt or animal fat. Avoid any animal food of any kind that is neither fish nor poultry. Note: There is growing insistence by nutritional therapists on the total avoidance of *all* animal protein, including fish and poultry.

Tea, Coffee: May be used moderately, but without any sweeteners, and generally should be avoided. Herb teas suggested as substitute. Note: Some clinicians emphasize a total avoidance of caffeinated coffee or anything with caffeine in it.

Tobacco: Should be strictly avoided.

Sweeteners: Should not be added to any food. The avoidance of refined sugar and products containing refined sugar is essential.

In terms of hygiene, the booklet recommends that patients not remain in a room with a smoker, that they increase their oxygen intake with exercises in the open air and away from known sources of pollution, that they take daily warm baths, evacuate their bowels at least once a day, sleep "adequately," avoid permanent-wave lotions, toxic hair sprays, synthetic cosmetics, antiperspirants and lipsticks made out of coal-tar dyes, and view television "as little as possible."

The last is in response to studies indicating that small doses of X-irradiation cause abnormal activity in plant and animal cells and that X-irradiation dosages are in fact cumulative.

Throughout the therapy, patients are given urine tests for the presence of the human chorionic gonadotropin (HCG) hormone.

When a "cancer crisis" has been successfully controlled for more than two years, with patients showing good objective responses in weight gain, increased strength, return to a more nearly normal state of activity and vigor, exhibiting negative HCG tests and showing an improvement in X-rays or other objective evidence, the maintenance of B-17 may be reduced to "dietary levels" of nitriloside of at least 500 milligrams per day.

The McNaughton handbook states that "there are no contraindications to the use of vitamin B-17 and/or the proteolytic enzymes along with surgery, radiation, and the cytotoxins." Hence, as the National Cancer Institute's Dr. Dean Burk has consistently pointed out, there is no good reason why a cancer patient may not take Laetrile along with other therapy.

The various practitioners around the world approach their overall Laetrile therapy differently, anxious to blend the best possible results from the known forms of cancer therapy. Dr. Hans Nieper of West Germany is by no means exclusively a "Laetrile doctor" — he simply has used amygdalin successfully in a variety of cases along with other treatments. Nor are Dr. Contreras, his doctors and the Clinica Cydel staff in Tijuana exclusively "Laetrile" doctors. They use amygdalin either as a treatment of choice in metabolic therapy or simply as another chemotherapeutic agent — one that is not toxic — in conjunction with "orthodox" therapies. But Dr. Krebs, McNaughton and other Laetrile "purists" would insist that, other than in the case of selective surgery, radiation and chemotherapy could and should usually be avoided altogether. It is McNaughton's dream for metabolic therapy and holistic medicine that cancer will eventually be resolved first through total metabolic means, in which vitamin B-17 is the crown jewel in a multivitamin treatment diadem, and that cancer will then be prevented altogether through diet — and through the mind.

The McNaughton handbook states the laetrilist position on surgery, radiotherapy, and chemotherapy, the approved approaches to cancer control, this way:

> *All forms of radiation can in one degree or another shrink benign as well as neoplastic tumors. Many of the cancer chemotherapeutic agents are similarly capable of shrinking tumors, malignant or benign. Unfortunately any shrinkage is gained at [the] cost of destroying somatic cells, especially the primitive repair cells.*
>
> *Although many benign tumors are radio-sensitive, and while the trophoblast growths of the chorionepitheliomas and similarly highly malignant undifferentiated cells are radio-resistant, the radiation may increase the proportion of neoplastic cells in the tumor, making the index of tumefaction a misleading and unreliable criterion of antineoplastic therapeutic response.*
>
> *However, surgery is often life-saving in cancer by correcting blockages, repairing fistulas, correcting hemorrhage, reconstructing plastic damage, and the like.*
>
> *If surgery can remove a tumor completely, as in early non-metastatic cancer of the uterus, it may conserve the health and life of the patient. The same applies to the use of surgery in preneoplastic hyperplasias, and polyps, papillomata, skin lesions, leukoplakia, senile keratoses, etc. Where rational surgery is used, B-17 and proteolytic enzyme therapy is not contraindicated in any way, and is indicated even before surgery.*
>
> *Since pulmonary neoplasms appear to be especially responsive to the use of vitamin B-17 and proteolytic enzymes, such an approach is the preferred method of treatment.*
>
> *Except for lesions in or close to the skin, radiation or the radiomimetic cytotoxins are to be avoided because of their highly immunosuppressive and other destructive effects.[4]*

The general megavitamin therapy experience of Doctors Richardson and McDonald, in California and Georgia, respectively, involves avoidance of chemotherapy and radiation. Other clinicians occasionally mixed these "orthodox" forms with the Laetrile-based vitamin therapy. The general consensus of every practioner I talked to was that advanced cancer cases previously treated with these customary approaches made the "control" aspects of Laetrile more difficult. The fact that the vast majority of American patients who ultimately turned to Laetrile (whether from Contreras, Nieper, Richardson, McDonald, or anyone else) were already described as "terminal" patients greatly clouded the efficacy of Laetrile as a "control" — for, as stated, no claims were made that Laetrile therapy could restore lost or damaged tissue.

Dr. McDonald's one-year experience with Laetrile and megavitamin therapy in Georgia convinced him, he told me, that all eighty of his patients had shown palliative symptoms from the Laetrile-vitamin approach, particularly decrease in pain, renewed appetite, and an extended life span. "So many who come in are at the point of death, after extreme radiation and chemotherapy. Chemotherapy seems to be worse than radiation — it really knocks the body for a loop," he said.

McDonald, who went on to become a U.S. Congressman and an able defender of "freedom of choice" at the federal level, added that it had been his brief experience that patients who had the best response to Laetrile therapy were at the time cancer-free but had had a past history of malignancies. The phrase "I've never felt better in my life" summarized their response to metabolic therapy.

The Atlanta urologist, once skeptical of Laetrile and learning of the details of Laetrile therapy and the trophoblast theory at a San Francisco seminar, also said:

> I had heard of trophoblast, but never the trophoblast concept. American doctors get no instruction in nutrition. No wonder American medicine has a blind spot. We generally are taught to believe the American diet is the best, that the stable American diet is good in nutrition. Sure, we get filled and people look happy, but that shouldn't be confused with nutrition.
>
> Medical schools simply do not teach nutrition. I had no nutrition in four years of medical school — oh, I guess one lecture, but I was out delivering a baby at that time.

From the new wave of treatment, investigation, and open — if "illegal" — use of Laetrile in the United States, and from information continuing to come in from around the world, came the most tantalizing of possibilities, quite in line with biochemist Ernst T. Krebs, Jr.'s dream: In nutrition lies not only "control" of cancer, but very likely its prevention.

CHAPTER FIFTEEN

The Case Against Laetrile — And Hope for the Future

THE CASE AGAINST LAETRILE, whether advanced by the Food and Drug Administration, the American Medical Association, the American Cancer Society, or state departments of public health, includes these elements, each and every one of them disputed in whole or part by Krebs, Burk, and the Laetrile physicians around the world:

• That sufficient case data on clinical use of Laetrile have not been brought forward.

• That the existing data on Laetrile show it to be of no real effect in combating cancer. Ditto the urine test for the detection of cancer through HCG release.

• That the real danger in Laetrile use, aside from veiled references to its cyanide action, is that the individual who turns to it will frequently do so in lieu of recognized or orthodox treatment.

• That the chemistry claimed in Laetrile action is not necessarily consistent with what actually happens in the body; that is, the Krebs premises do not actually hold up.

Then, of course, the inferences that can be drawn from the FDA and related actions against Laetrile and the Laetrile-bearing products "Bee Seventeen" and "Aprikern," and even against apricot kernels themselves, are even more alarming to the layman. Since the admitted active in-gredient in the Laetrile attack on cancer is cyanide, and cyanide is a poison, then, *ipso facto*, Laetrile and Laetrile-bearing products are dangerous.

The rationales advanced to explain "control" claims of Laetrile-using patients, and often put to me by representatives of "orthodoxy," are these:

• The individual in question may never have had cancer in the first place.

• If he is responding well now, or seems to respond well now, it may be because he is finally responding to the orthodox treatments he received earlier.

• The individual may have undergone "spontaneous remission" of symptoms.

To update myself as much as possible on the "case" against Laetrile, I asked the American Cancer Society a number of specifics. The answers, researched and relayed to me very kindly by Charles Dahle, director of public information, American Cancer Society, California Division, included the following:

Questioned as to whether the ACS has sponsored research into nutritional or vitamin factors in the possible prevention or treatment of cancer: "In recent years the American Cancer Society has not sponsored research into nutritional or vitamin factors in the possible prevention or treatment of cancer, primarily because no applications from scientists have been received.

"There have been a few scattered projects of this kind in earlier years, but these have been mainly epidemiological. Most research touching on nutritional factors has been epidemiological. It is my understanding that it has uncovered no significant dietary factors relating to cancer."

Questioned as to whether ACS has attempted to investigate the claims made by proponents of Laetrile, particularly after 1963, and if not, why not: "... The Society has been unable since 1963 to fund more than a portion of the scientifically approved research applications it has received. Unfortunately, claims made for Laetrile have not stood up under scientific scrutiny. Since investigations of this product have been adequately carried out by others, nothing would be gained by diverting funds for the purpose of going back over old ground.

"It is my understanding that since 1963 the California State Department of Health has been most receptive to the making of studies on Laetrile, but that its efforts in this direction have been hampered by failure of Laetrile proponents to supply verified case histories for examination ..."

Questioned as to amount of money raised by the Cancer Society in its annual fund drives and how they are allocated: "During its 1971-72 fiscal year the American Cancer Society received a total of approximately $79 million in contributions and legacies. The allocation of these funds for the 1972-73 budget can be considered typical, and will be found on page 29 of *Cancer Facts & Figures*. During the 1972-73 fiscal year the Society received approximately $93 million in contributions and legacies."

This figure had reached $107 million in 1975, and the last reported budget (for 1974-75) in 1976 *Cancer Facts and Figures* was $99.8 million dollars, with approximately $28 million spent either on "public and professional education," a whopping $11.9 million for fund raising, about $10 million for "management and general," aside from $29 million for "research." The list of grants mentioned predominantly was for continuing work in buttressing the viral theory of cancer. A few, however, did reflect some interest in studying immune defense mechanisms — a move viewed by metabolic physicians as at least a mini-step in the right direction.

I was intrigued by the amounts spent not only for "research" but also for "education" — for, if there were just a shadow of a glimmer of an insinuation that Laetrile *might* be effective, if only as an analgesic, why not a tiny little effort in that direction? At the same time, the ACS had unleashed a campaign of attack on cancer quackery and had placed Laetrile at the top of the "quackery" list. Its spokesmen (and spokeswomen) continued to repeat the hoary falsehood that there is not a "shred of evidence" for Laetrile's efficacy. It was impossible, of course, to detect how much of the budget for "education" went into pooh-poohing Laetrile.

Questioned as to the cost of cancer to individual patients: "Information on the cost of cancer to individual patients is difficult to compile because of the varying nature of the disease and the treatment it requires. Averages, therefore, would not be too meaningful even if they were available." I was referred to *Cancer Facts & Figures* as to cancer costs.

My interest here was trying to track down facts and figures to support or demolish the claims that cancer represents a mammoth industry worth billions of dollars. One source, *California Business* for November 9, 1972, had indicated upwards of $12 billion per year cost, based on an estimated median expenditure per cancer patient. I had variously heard the amounts a cancer patient ultimately pays during the entire course of therapy estimated at ranges of anywhere from $13,000 to $30,000, much more in many cases, less in others.

The unofficially reported increase of the cost of cancer treatment for terminal patients of $30,000 and more, and the cost of the considerable increase in both cancer incidence and fatalities, were not reflected in the ACS *Facts and Figures* data between 1974 and 1976, which stuck with a treatment-and-related figure of $3 billion per year (a figure forthcoming from an ACS conference in 1972), but added that "if direct and indirect costs of cancer (loss of productivity, earning power) are added, the estimated figure would jump to a national bill of $15 billion." This was $10 billion less than the tab estimated by governmental sources, but nonetheless reflected the enormous cost of cancer (and, we daresay, of profits *from* cancer).

Questioned as to whether the American Cancer Society has a controlling interest, in, or substantial patents on, the chemotherapy drug 5-FU fluorouracil (This point was frequently raised by laetrilists to suggest such a link between the ACS and one of the heavily toxic "drugs of choice" that a vested interest in the society to oppose a relatively simple — let alone inexpensive — answer to cancer might be inferred.): "The American Cancer

Society frequently has been libeled and slandered about alleged profits received from patents on anti-cancer drugs.

"The only patent held by the American Cancer Society is for the drugs 5-FU and 5-FUDR. The Society's ownership consists of ½ of ½ of an undivided interest. The owner of the other ½ of ½ of undivided interest is the U.S. government.

"The Society ownership rights were held to guarantee that opportunities would be provided for licensing and manufacturing these drugs in the event that other owners of the patent decided not to make it available to the public. This eventuality did not occur and is no longer considered a possibility, because the drugs are now in common use. At no time has the Society profited from cancer, nor does it expect to. No royalties have been received or are payable to the Society or any of its Divisions."

The ACS's official position on Laetrile had not changed at all since I first read it in 1971: "After careful study of the literature and other information available to it, the American Cancer Society does not have evidence that treatment with Laetrile results in objective benefit in the treatment of cancer in human beings." Again, the California studies on Laetrile are the basis on which the prohibitions against interstate shipment of Laetrile and conclusions of worthlessness were ultimately based.

The 1953 California Cancer Commission report, with its ambivalent wording and low stated dosages on forty-four patients, and the lack of familiarity of any of the members of the commission with the substance, was followed by a report ten years later that in essence repeated the conclusions of the 1953 report. A supplemental report to that one followed in 1966, based on fourteen clinical records submitted by the Mc-Naughton Foundation and the North End Medical Center, both in Montreal, Quebec. "These were not complete records but were abstracts furnished by the various hospitals in Canada to the McNaughton Foundation," stated the California Cancer Advisory Council's preface.

This supplemental report found that the clinical studies, variously describing types of palliation from Laetrile, were "inadequate." It also included a *Canadian Medical Association Journal* study which cast doubt on the chemical mechanism claimed by laetrilists.[1] It was dealing with two varieties of the substance then being manufactured.

At the federal level, the National Cancer Institute in Bethesda, Maryland, reported in 1960 that it had tested Laetrile on mice with transplanted tumors with negative results. In subsequent animal tests at NCI, the fact that varying experts could reach opposite conclusions as to the effectiveness of Laetrile on mouse tumors is best demonstrated by the one-man battle of the NCI cytochemistry chief, Dr. Dean Burk, who argued that tests on mice *did* demonstrate the effectiveness of the substance. His statistical analyses of the several NCI animal studies with Laetrile reached conclusions opposite to those put forth by the governmental body. He was also outspoken in his detailed assessment of the early, but mixed, results of the Sloan-Kettering tests.

So the rigidity at the federal government level regarding Laetrile remained as unyielding as the position adopted by the ACS. In explaining why "funds are no longer allocated" to evaluate Laetrile, inquiries to the National Cancer Institute as late as 1975 were still apt to be referred to the same statement made by the NCI to Rep. James C. Cleveland in April 1973: "In order to resolve the conflicting reports obtained in experiments with laboratory animals, the National Cancer Institute over recent months has again conducted tests of Laetrile, both alone and in combination with beta-glucosidase in a variety of experimental tumor systems," read the letter from the NCI acting director. "No evidence of reproducible anti-tumor activity has been found. Inasmuch as the Institute has now completed its testing of Laetrile, funds are no longer allocated for evaluation of this drug."

That conclusion, of course, directly contradicts the findings of Dr. Burk and inferentially contradicts the findings of some of the Sloan-Kettering tests. Nonetheless, such conclusive rejections constituted the official position on Laetrile.

In 1974, while preparing the first version of this book, I sought a demonstrably effective rebuttal to Laetrile — one that had been successfully answered by the Laetrile proponents. Surely, I thought, California state authorities might have on hand (a) an example of a continual Laetrile user who had never at any time received, or even thought he received, any benefits from use of the substance; (b) a solid case of a patient whose premature death from cancer could demonstrably be linked to dependence on Laetrile to the exclusion of the standard treatments; or (c) a solid case of near fatality or other demonstrated severe toxicity from Laetrile use. It's true that my probe was a telephone one. Nonetheless, the *best* evidence suggested to me by public health officials was the 1953 test results.

As indicated, the 1953 results constitute only the thinnest and most superficial attack on Laetrile — it is a very weak argument, indeed, on which to base persistent refusals to move ahead with officially sanctioned tests on humans in 1976. But the official positions and statements remained unchanged, as far as organized, orthodox medicine was concerned. Laetrile, at least officially, was taboo. Any mention of it in professional circles usually sparked an emotional response. With a cancer death rate achieving a record high in the United States, it was understandably difficult to approach the epidemic of cancer with other than a display of emotionalism.

Any suggestion that Laetrile might hold the key to a solution was certain to get a sharp rejection from outstanding specialists. Jesse Steinfeld, the former U.S. surgeon general who also had been a member of the California Cancer Advisory Committee, and whose early denunciation of Laetrile was the ever-recurring basis for subsequent actions against it, was still saying: "There just were not any anti-tumor effects (from tests on Laetrile). It's been tested and retested over the years without success."

He was quoted, along with Mayo Clinic specialist Dr. David Carr, in the *Rochester* (Minn.) *Post-Bulletin*, the daily newspaper in the Mayo Clinic's hometown. Between January 21-25, 1974, the newspaper joined the small but growing number of publications that had done in-depth studies of Laetrile. The *Post-Bulletin* quoted Carr: "There is just no valid scientific evidence that Laetrile checks cancer."

The newspaper, however, interviewed numerous Minnesota-area Laetrile users, among the hundreds of Minnesotans who had joined the thousands of Americans making the trip to Tijuana in 1973. As in my own Bay Area interviews, the *Post-Bulletin* interviews produced a consistent report of positive results from Laetrile users, ranging from relief of pain to actual regression of tumors. The newspaper also turned up rigid refusals by authorities and cancer specialists to acknowledge any of these testimonials.

As a California State Public Health Department spokesman had told me on several occasions: "Any quack cure can turn up testimonials. We're not interested in testimonials. We want solid medical case histories." Although I did indeed see several sets of credible medical case histories, there was no single, solid set of documents that would apparently meet the criteria demanded by officialdom: diagnoses of cancer made in the United States by reputable physicians, with treatment by Laetrile (and its ancillary therapy) only and exclusively from the onset of the symptoms.

But by 1976, not only had such cases as Glen Rutherford fulfilled such requirements, but they were beginning to be made known to organizations like the Committee for Freedom of Choice in Cancer Therapy, Inc., in ever-greater numbers. Increasingly, patients with sound diagnoses and treated *solely* with Laetrile and its ancillary therapy were becoming available. Yet these, as in all cases before them, were cavalierly waved aside as "anecdotal."

The vast majority of Laetrile patients remained those already adjudged terminal — literally given up for dead — by medical orthodoxy. This meant that before turning to the apricot kernel they had, in the great majority of cases, already been treated with chemotherapy, radiation, or surgery, or a combination of all three. What happened to them afterward could be applauded or decried by orthodoxy depending on the outcome. Although experienced clinicians around the world had dealt with thousands of Laetrile patients, their data and reports were simply unacceptable to American orthodoxy.

In California, birthplace of the Laetrile research and development, statements by California officials continued to suggest that not only is Laetrile worthless, but, because of its cyanide action, it may have a toxicity factor. In an American Cancer Society statement circulated in 1973 and entitled *Questions and Answers on Quackery*, Grant Leake, program supervisor of the California Food and Drug Section fraud unit, and Dr. Ralph Weilerstein, former executive secretary of the California Cancer Advisory Council, reserved their harshest attacks for Laetrile. Dr. Weilerstein stated:

> *The number of quacks may be decreasing, but I see a marked increase in the well-organized promotion of certain quack remedies, primarily Laetrile. This promotion seems rather skillful, uses up-to-date advertising and public relations techniques, and makes excellent use of the media. Hiding behind the constitutional guarantees of freedom of speech and freedom of the press, the quack promoters are getting their message across.*

Stating that, as to Laetrile testimonials, "absolutely none . . . has ever been proven," he added, "We know that many persons who give testimonials never had cancer. Others had orthodox treatment in addition to a quack remedy and, although they are more than willing to swear that it was a quack remedy that helped them, it was no doubt the surgery, radiation or chemotherapy."

Moreover, he repeated in the officially sanctioned "questions and answers": "Over the past 20 years there have been animal studies, chemical studies, review of theory and extensive reviews by medical groups and the courts of case histories submitted by the proponents. Laetrile's proponents admit that it's been given to thousands of persons. And yet they cannot produce even one medically substantiated case which shows any beneficial effects — not one."

In the same document, Leake warns:

> *Be suspicious of anyone who talks of secret cures, of persecution by the "medical establishment," who makes a difficult diagnosis on the first examination, or warns against consulting another physician. The charge of a worldwide conspiracy to keep a cancer cure under wraps just doesn't hold water. Doctors, researchers and their families die of cancer too. If they knew of any cure, they'd use it. These so-called remedies are not used on the other side of the Iron Curtain either, so how can it be a profit-making plot?*

Remarks as to "not even one medically substantiated case" were simply in total error by 1976, yet they were consistently and continually repeated by the American Medical Association, the American Cancer Society, the National Cancer Institute, the Food and Drug Administration, and state boards of medical health and state medical societies.

While the honest intent of the above statements is unquestioned, the inferences to be drawn from them left me with unanswered questions. Just as a terminal cancer patient seemingly undergoing partial or total control of his disease cannot with total certainty claim that Laetrile is the reason for the control, by no means can orthodox medicine with total certainty make the claim that such control is the result of the delayed success of surgery, radiation, or chemotherapy. The remarks about doctors and their families, of course, skirted the reality that a growing number of physicians in the States *do* use Laetrile.

Clearly, officialdom and medical orthodoxy are hedging on the question of Laetrile. I do not wish to indicate I believe they are hedging because of a binding, monolithic conspiracy, however much vested interests undoubtedly and inevitably do play a role. The people who make up officialdom and medical orthodoxy are, after all, only human beings, equipped with a full range of strengths and weaknesses. But ego concerns and entrenched attitudes, whether they are based on false premises or not, are also clearly evident in the American cancer tragedy. Nobody wants to say, "I was wrong." It is, in a sense, insulting to the modern medical mind to be told, for example, that cancer is simply a vitamin-deficiency disease and that it may be prevented by a treatment no more complicated than adequate diet.

Nor do I hurl criticism at rank-and-file physicians and rank-and-file bureaucrats. They — we — all tend to follow the leader. We all seek a certain amount of refuge in the known, the presumably demonstrated, the safely orthodox. It is certainly no crime to behave in this distinctly human fashion.

Again, while I do not denounce officialdom and orthodoxy as part of a gigantic conspiracy — venal, evil beings meeting together to plot the next operation aimed at making the human race sicker — I certainly cannot (and I believe no journalist can) take the opposite stance: that the growing wave of Laetrile testimonials come from people who don't know what they're talking about, people who either never had cancer in the first place or are responding to some previous orthodox treatment; that those involved in Laetrile are a sideshow of kooks, freaks, criminals, extremists, and sundry fanatics (however much fanaticism and some extremism may occassionally be present); that responsible scientists, doctors, and researchers around the world who have been involved with Laetrile in various stages of its development and advance are parts either of a criminal conspiracy or of a mutual admiration team of pseudoscientists; and that, ultimately, Laetrile is a giant, sinister con game whose target is the growing number of terminal cancer patients virtually abandoned by modern science.

That Laetrile may soon be vindicated in the United States, after almost a quarter century of suppression, and that Krebs may be right about the nature and prevention of cancer — these developments, should they occur, will be testimonials to an ever-recurring reality in human events and nature itself: the answer to complicated problems is often simplicity itself.

Established powers clearly are being dishonest in focusing on such aspects of Laetrile as ad-hominem attacks on Krebs and McNaughton, the presence of Birch Society members (or any other elements deemed "undesirable") in the Laetrile cause, or by overly emphasizing the controversy about the focal action of Laetrile or the assault on its presumptive vitamin status. None of these attacks deals with the real issues involved.

If there were simply a *hint* of Laetrile efficacy in the prevention, treatment, alleviation or management of cancer, or in the relief of cancer-related pain, then there is no sound or moral reason for Laetrile to be "banned" — particularly when both the incidence of cases of cancer and fatalities from cancer are at an all-time high and when "orthodox" therapies are so miserably failing to dent those statistics.

Next (and this is perhaps the more vital of the issues), by what moral right does the state interfere in the doctor-patient relationship in blocking access *by both* to an alternative therapy, particularly when the patient already has been judged "terminal" and incurable by orthodox medicine?

It is the failure to answer, in any convincing way, this last question which has shifted the onus of guilt onto the established powers. In the name of justice, in the name of humanity, how long must vitamin B-17 remain illegal?

The revelations of the Watergate era and such followup scandals as the Lockheed bribery brought into increasing question the morality and honesty of government and its overlap with vested interests. One need not be paranoid to fear the combined forces of the international pharmaceutical cartel and the food-processing industry may very well exert such enormous pressure on the expanding police powers of government so as to advance wanted substances and wanted legislation and to block unwanted substances and unwanted legislation.

For we can make no mistake about it:

A medical revolution looms on the horizon in the "civilized" world, a world plagued not by the infectious and parasitic diseases of old, but by the degenerative killer diseases of today — and the evidence is growing exponentially that these diseases are interlocking parts of a whole, that the whole is involved with metabolic breakdown, and that the primary influencing factor in metabolic breakdown is diet. Man *has* strayed from biological sanity and millions of years of evolutionary reality through the wholesale alteration of his diet in the last few thousand years. This is particularly noticeable in the "civilized" countries, where basic, whole, natural foods have been replaced by denaturalized simulations divested of their vitamins, artificially colored or padded for visual effect; loaded with artificial flavorings and preservatives; and treated with everything from bleaches, texture enhancers, dough conditioners and softeners to antifoamers, sweeteners, emulsifiers, and other substances in the name of "enrichment." The price "civilized" man is paying for his departure from biological sanity is a runaway epidemic of degenerative disease, in which the worst forms — heart disease and cancer — are now the major killers of the industrialized world.

The challenge is *not* being met by "crisis medicine" — by medicine as usual. It is not being met by pouring billions of dollars into the research and development of new and more powerful toxic drugs and their combinations, or by graduating more knife-wielding surgical experts. It is not being met by building gleaming new clinics and prohibitively costly hospitals, or the whole conglomerate of enterprises euphemistically advertised as "health-care delivery."

While human technology expands at a geometric rate, and runs roughshod over nature in the process, we may very well have overlooked a number of simple solutions to the problems that beset us. This will probably turn out to be true about energy, pollution, and diminishing natural resources, and doubtless will be true in medicine. The nation that consumes billions of pills per year for virtually every affliction, real or imagined, is a nation with a runaway cancer epidemic and growing statistics to indicate that that nation is getting sicker, not healthier. Surely, something is wrong somewhere. In medicine in general and cancer in particular, surely something, something very crucial, has been overlooked. The answer may be so simple as to be staring us in the face.

This "something" may very well be that cancer arises as a natural part of the life cycle, runs unchecked only because of man's uninformed and unintentional tampering with that cycle, and surely has a natural use and inhibitor within that life cycle. This may be true — it probably *is* true — for virtually every disease. There is nothing naturally malignant in the universe, insists Ernst Krebs, Jr. This is a profoundly religious statement.

Much may be gained by returning to biological sanity — and to some of the simple dictates of lifestyle enshrined in the Bible. Strangely enough, the medical revolution, carrying with it in no small part a back-to-nature kind of aura, will be a *return* to preventive medicine, a *return* to the ancient concepts of dealing with the whole man rather than treating a specific disease.

Thomas A. Edison foresaw precisely this situation when he said: "The doctor of the future will give no medicine but will interest his patients in the care of the human frame, in diet, and in the cause and prevention of disease."

And the ultimate importance of *mind* in therapy will be a big part — if not the *major* part — of the coming medical revolution.

It is Dr. Dennis Myers of San Francisco, I believe, who summed it up best. Perhaps a harbinger of a new wave of medical men who think in terms of a universal, organic totality, he made this the slogan of his medical practice:

"Dis-ease is a contradiction with God. It begins in the Mind which passes it to the feeling nature. This feeling body can manifest it as a neurosis or a psychosis or can pass it on to the physical form where it will manifest as a physical ailment. Diagnosis is intuitive and simple. Treatment consists simply of responding to the situation with sincerity. The situation reveals the cure, when it is Time."

FOOTNOTES

CHAPTER ONE

1. The claim by Laetrilists that vitamin B-17 is "legal" in two dozen other countries has been called into question by American orthodoxy. The facts are that Laetrile has been legally shipped to, or used in, two dozen countries without legal interference from their governments, since in most of these countries it is *not* incumbent on governmental edict to "legalize" a drug. The countries which, as of 1976, had allowed shipments of personal use of Laetrile, or had allowed its use experimentally, are: Argentina, Australia (now allowable for patient use and shipped through the Ministry of Health), Brazil, China (mainland), East Germany (used in amygdalin experiments), Estonia, France, Great Britain, Greece, Indonesia (being used clinically and experimentally both from local and foreign sources), Italy, Lebanon (shipped for evaluation experiments), Mexico (specifically legal as an analgesic in lung cancer and under evaluation), Monte Carlo (site of a Laetrile-producing facility), Nicaragua, Peru, Philippines (experimentally and clinically used and reported on at Univeristy of Santo Tomas Research Center despite no *de jure* legal status by the government), Poland, the Soviet Union, Spain, Switzerland, Venezuela, West Germany (legal for general use as "activated amygdalin"), and Yugoslavia. In no country is Laetrile under any name a "drug of choice" in cancer therapy. (Data from The McNaughton Foundation.)

2. Daniel S. Greenberg, "Cancer: Now the Bad News," *Journal of the International Academy of Preventive Medicine*, Second Quarter 1975. Appeared earlier in the *Columbia Journalism Review* and *Washington Post*.

3. In *Midnight*, September 1, 1975, and abstracted in "Cancer 'treatments' hasten death: Jones," THE CHOICE (official publication of The Committee for Freedom of Choice in Cancer Therapy, Inc.) October 1975.

4. From The *National Enquirer* and abstracted in "Cancer and Vitamin 'A' Deficiency," THE CHOICE, April 1976.

5. Nicholas Gonzalez, "Preventing," *Family Health/Today's Health*, May 1976.

6. Joseph L. Lyon, M.D., M.P.H.; Melville R. Klauber, Ph.D.; John W. Gardner, M.S.; and Charles R. Smart, M.D., in *New England Journal of Medicine*, January 15, 1976, and abstracted in "Puzzle: less cancer among Mormons," THE CHOICE, April 1976.

7. Jack Anderson column abstracted in "U.S. falling behind in nutrition-cancer research," THE CHOICE, April 1976.

CHAPTER TWO

1. Food and Drug Administration spokesmen have stated that there is no sngle regulation which "bans" the interstate shipment and sale of Laetrile, and that the FDA considers the assertion there is such a ban "unfortunate." However, the FDA statement of September 1, 1971, reporting on consultants' findings on Laetrile, reads in part: "Under the FDA position reinforced today by the Ad Hoc Committee findings, Laetrile (amygdalin) may not be promoted, tested, or sold in the United States under

provisions of the Federal Food, Drug and Cosmetic Act until the necessary basic studies have been accomplished." The FDA points out that *no* product which has not been cleared for an Investigative New Drug (IND) order may be so sold or shipped. Laetrile falls into this category, but there is no specific anti-Laetrile regulation. Hence there *is* a ban against it, though not a specific one, and more than one attorney has questioned whether FDA statements and general regulations constitutionally have the force of law.

2. Ernst T. Krebs, Jr. "The Nitrilosides (Vitamin B-17) — Their Nature, Occurrence and Metabolic Significance." *Journal of Applied Nutrition* 22, nos. 3, 4 (1970).

3. Copy of letter with the author.

4. Barbara J. Culliton, "Sloan-Kettering: The Trials of an Apricot Pit — 1973," *Science* (December 1, 1973).

5. Brian Sullivan, *Associated Press*, February 4, 1974.

6. *Anatomy of a Coverup: Successful Sloan-Kettering Amygdalin (Laetrile) Animal Studies.* The Committee for Freedom of Choice in Cancer Therapy, Inc., Los Altos, California, 1975.

7. "Laetrile Testing: A Coverup that Wasn't," *Medical World News*, October 6, 1975.

8. David Rorvik. "Laetrile: The Goddamned-Contraband-Apricot Connection," newsletter, The Alicia Patterson Foundation, New York, July 1976.

9. "A Critical Evaluation of Cancer Chemotherapy," *Cancer Research* Vol. 29, pp. 2262-69.

10. P.G. Reitnauer, in *Arch. Geschwulstforsch* 42, no. 4 (1974): 135-37.

11. Memorandum and statement from National Cancer Institute, dated December 19, 1973.

12. *Ibid.*, dated October 26, 1973.

CHAPTER THREE

1. Letter made available to the author.

2. Letter made available to the author.

3. *Affidavit in Support of Motion for Order Staying Execution of Sentence.* People vs. Eli von Pinoci *et al.* California Superior Court, San Diego, Case. No. CR. 32978. February 9, 1976.

4. George Browne, Jr., D.V.M., "Remission of Canine Thyroid Carcinoma Following Nitriloside Therapy." *Veterinary Medicine/Small Animal Clinician*, February 1974.

CHAPTER FOUR

1. Raymond Crawfurd, *The Last Days of Charles II* (Oxford: Clarendon Press, 1909).

2. Drs. Sidney J. Cutler and Lester Breslow in February 1976 set the 1974 "national bill for all health care" at $100 billion, a conservative figure which undoubtedly did not include all ramifications of the "health-care delivery industry." They estimated an expense of $4 to $5 billion for cancer care, again a figure probably far short of the entire expense (and profit) involved in cancer.

3. Morris A. Bealle, *Super Drug Story* (Washington: Columbia Publishing Co., 1962).

4. Reported in *San Francisco Examiner*, April 29, 1976.

5. Alan Stang, "Laetrile: Freedom of Choice in Cancer Therapy?" *American Opinion*, January 1974.

CHAPTER FIVE

1. Quoted in Adelaide Hechtlinger, *The Great Patent Medicine Era* (New York: Grosset & Dunlap, 1970).

2. Herbert M. Summa, "Amygdalin: A Physiologically Active Therapeutic Agent in Malignancies," *Krebsgeschehen* 4 (1972). (Translated from the German.)

3. Krebs, Jr. discussed the vitamin B-17 theory in "The Nitrilosides (Vitamin B-17) — Their Nature, Occurrence and Metabolic Significance," *Journal of Applied Nutrition* 22, nos. 3, 4 (1970).

4. Cited by Wynn Westover, McNaughton Foundation, in *Summary of The McNaughton Foundation IND 6734 with Addenda*, 1973 (P.O. Box 853, Sausalito, California).

5. London: Chatto & Windus, 1911.

6. Dr. Charles Gurchot, Ernst Krebs' former teacher and a Beardian himself, notes that "it is only fair to say that non-Beardians would claim that the degeneration of the trophoblast is brought about by the increasing pressure on it" by the rapid growth of the fetus.

7. Ernst T. Krebs, Jr., Ernst T. Krebs, Sr., and Howard H. Beard, "The Unitarian or Trophoblastic Thesis of Cancer," *Medical Record* (July 1950).

8. Charles Gurchot, *Biology — The Key to the Riddle of Cancer* (New York: Moore Publishers, 1949).

9. In *Oncology*, Vol. 31, No. 5-6, 1975, Dr. Gurchot made an important new contribution to Beardianism. In "The Trophoblast Theory of Cancer (John Beard, 1857-1924) Revisited," he tackles a problem which followers of the theory have long puzzled over: Whether it is proper to say that cancer or trophoblast arise *only* from the aberrant primitive germ cells. Backed by 93 scientific papers and books, Dr. Gurchot demonstrates in the *Oncology* article that "cancer represents primarily trophoblastic tissue derived either from an aberrant germ cell *or from a somatic cell whose repressed 'asexual generation' genes are abnormally reactivated ('derepressed')." [Emphasis ours.]. This abnormal reactivation — or "de-repression" — may be brought about by the substances and conditions generally described as "carcinogenic" or cancer-causing, including certain chemicals, radiation, and toxic substances. Genetic information, including "asexual generation," is present in a somatic or normal cell, but this "information" is normally repressed. The activities of carcinogenesis may "de-repress" — that is, activate — such "information," and asexual generation (trophoblast, or cancer) may be the result. It is as if a computer "fed" with several inputs of information were adversely affected by a faulty switch or damage to the mechanism so that a computer program which the operator has not called for suddenly appears on the console — *i.e.*, the wrong "information" is coming out of the computer. As Gurchot writes of this updated Beardianism: "Although it represents a correction of Beard's general thesis, it also tends to validate his principal conclusion; namely, the role of trophoblast in cancer." Additionally, one would speculate that it still means the body's immunosuppressive system is going to continue to react to cancer (or trophoblast) the same way whether that cancer (or trophoblast) arises from an aberrant primitive germ cell or from normal cells.

10. Charles Oberling, *The Riddle of Cancer*, trans. Woglon (New Haven: Yale University Press, 1944).

CHAPTER SIX

1. Wynn Westover, "Listing of Documents Relative to the Krebs Enzyme Extracts Later Known as Laetrile," in *Summary of the McNaughton Foundation* IND 6734 (*April 6,*

FREEDOM FROM CANCER

1970-*February* 1971) with *Addenda*, McNaughton Foundation, P.O. Box 853, Sausalito, Calif., 1973.

2. Glenn Kittler, *Laetrile — Control for Cancer* (New York: Paperback Library, 1963).

3. San Francisco Vegetarian Society for Health and Humanity newsletter, January 1974.

4. Dr. Burk has also demonstrated a synergistic increase in antitumoral activity between the released hydrogen cyanide and benzaldehyde. The National Cancer Institute's cytochemistry division chief is nonetheless extremely careful about making conclusive statements as to the theoretical action of Laetrile, aside from its demonstrated chemical action. "Everybody usually appreciates it when I point out that old Charlie Chan statement: 'Charlie Chan say beware of theory — dew on eyeglasses can obscure fact,' " said Burk, doubtlessly taking some liberties with the inscrutable Oriental detective.

5. Part of the problem stems from the fact that not enough is known about the interaction of some specific enzymes. In his paper entitled "The Nitrilosides in Plants and Animals" (in *The Laetriles — Nitrilosides — in the Prevention and Control of Cancer*, a compilation by the McNaughton Foundation of vitamin B-17 papers on the vitamin's therapeutic implications), Dr. Krebs makes some educated suppositions about the action of Laetrile and suggests what might be the case with a synthetic Laetrile. His studies had already indicated the heavy (and indisputed) concentrations of the enzyme beta-glucuronidase, which is produced by the contiguous somatic cells in response to the presence of estrogen (estrogen being, again, the presumptive single stimulator for the division of a totipotent cell into a gametogenous cell with the consequential division into trophoblast). He states: "When the nitriloside . . . is parenterally (that is, outside the digestive system) administered as such it enters the bloodstream as an intact molecule. Malignant lesions are focally characterized by an especially high and selective concentration of beta-glucosidase and beta-glucuronidase. An extensive literature describes the high focal concentration of beta-glucuronidase that characterizes most malignant lesions. This concentration is often in excess of 300 times that of the contiguous somatic tissues. There is also a substantial literature describing the deficiency of the definitely malignant cell in rhodanese. The occurrence of beta-glucuronidase appears to be paralleled by an equal concentration of beta-glucosidase. Both enzymes are described generically as *beta-glycosidases*. Synthetic glucuronosidic nitrilosides (Laetrile) have been synthesized to exploit the beta-glucuronidase system in the same manner in which the natural nitrilosides are used against the beta-glucosidase system at the malignant lesion. In comparative studies it has been found that both the natural and synthetic nitrilosides are active against their respective enzyme systems." In a memorandum of March 18, 1972, to a Massachusetts Institute of Technology researcher, Krebs pointed out: "As you know, the natural nitriloside or Vitamin B-17 is a beta-glucoside. This is in itself not a target for beta-glucuronidase. We strongly suspect, however, that a beta-glucosidase system with an optimum pH (i.e., hydrogen ion concentration) below 6.0 is operative in neoplastic cells or tissues. Whether the same enzyme is also present but inactive at the lower hydrogen ion concentrations of the corresponding normal or somatic tissues — or whether the enzyme is unique to the neoplastic tissue — we do not know. I strongly favor the former hypothesis at this time."

6. Mark McCarty, "Burying Caesar: An Analysis of the Laetrile Problem," *Triton Times*, University of California at San Diego, November 29, 1975.

7. A Keith Brewer and Richard A. Passwater, "Physics of the cell membrane; mechanisms involved in cancer," Part V, *American Laboratory*, April 1976.

8. Their paper, "Tumor-selective Inhibition of Incorporation of 3H-Labeled Amino

Acids into Protein by Cyanate," was commented on extensively by Dr. Krebs, Jr. in THE CHOICE, November 1975.

9. Kittler, op. cit. — the source of the early (1950-53) descriptions of Laetrile therapy.

CHAPTER SEVEN

1. Dean Burk, letter to Rep. Louis Frey, Jr., May 30, 1972.

2. "Unproven Methods of Cancer Management — Laetrile," *Ca — A Cancer Journal for Clinicians* (American Cancer Society) July-August 1972.

3. Jim Dean and Frank Martinez, "The Laetrile Story," *Santa Ana Register*, October 4-9, 1964.

4. "The Treatment of Cancer with 'Laetriles,'" *California Medicine* 78, no. 4 (April 1953).

5. Letter, George Kell to R. K. Procunier, director, California Adult Authority, regarding prisoner Harvey E. Howard, October 16, 1973.

6. Walter S. Ross, "The Medicines We Need — But Can't Have," *Reader's Digest*, October 1973.

7. M. Stanton Evans, "Government Can Be Hazardous to Your Health," *Imprimis*, Hillside College, Hillsdale, Michigan. Vol. 4 No. 6, June 1975.

8. "Nation's Metabolic Experts Make Case for Legalization of California Chelation Therapy," *The Choice*, May 1976.

9. American Association of Medical Preventics (AAMP) testimony before California Medical Association ad hoc committee, Los Angeles, CA, March 26, 1976.

10. In contrast with the 17,000 per year mentioned in the *Rochester* (Minn.) *Post-Bulletin* series of January 21-25, 1974, an otherwise excellent account of the Laetrile story. Several thousand more visitors over the border above and beyond the 1,000 new patients per year may be explained by "repeaters" returning for Laetrile supplies.

11. Everett R. Holles, "Cancer Drug Smuggled into the USA," *Moneysworth*, May 10, 1976.

12. *Reporte Preliminar: Comprendido de 500 Casos de Pacientes Tratados con Laetrile-Amigdalina.* Dr. Ernesto Contreras R., Tijuana, Mexico, 1967.

13. Don C. Matchan, "A New Look at Laetrile," *Let's Live*, June 1973.

14. Statement before the House Subcommittee on Intergovernmental Operations.

15. Albert Segaloff, M.D., director, endocrine research, Alton Oschner Foundation, New Orleans; Melvin J. Krant, M.D., director, medical cancer unit, Tufts University, Medford, Mass.; David P. Rall, M.D., Ph.D., associate science director for experimental therapeutics, National Institute of Environmental Health Sciences, North Carolina; Michael B. Shimkin, M.D., professor of community medicine and oncology, University of California, San Diego; Julian L. Ambrus, M.D., Ph.D., director of cancer research, Roswell Park Memorial Institute, Buffalo, N.Y.

16. To Tom Valentine, *National Tattler*, March 11, 1973.

17. *The Choice*, May 1976. Dr. Soto called his program "CAP" — *i.e.*, 9 grams daily of amygdalin, along with 800 mg. of Cyclophosphamide and 80 mg. of Prednisone. The "CAP" treatment, he said, seemed to eliminate the usual toxic side effects associated with the latter two substances, while allowing them to work with amygdalin (Laetrile) against cancer. Dr. Ernst T. Krebs, Jr. strongly rebutted the theory of "mixed" toxic and nontoxic therapy (*The Choice*, May and June, 1976), arguing that the short-term gains which may result from a sudden diminution in the size of tumors is a false

criterion for measuring cancer therapy and that a "metabolic time bomb" has been set ticking by the use of cytotoxins which are poisonous to the body. Still, results of the "mixed" approach, at least in the short term, were impressive. The arguments of metabolic therapists against the use of tumor size as a criterion for gauging the results of cancer therapy are these: cancer tumors are local manifestations of a systemic or metabolic disease rather than a disease in and of themselves; the bigger cancerous tumors are, the more they are composed of normal, rather than malignant, tissue; hence, since cytotoxins and radiation destroy all tissues, it is to be expected that they will destroy much of the tumor mass — but whether they destroy actual cancer tissue remains the question. A sudden diminution of tumor size while the body's immune system is being attacked by poison represents "fool's gold" in cancer therapy, Krebs *et al* argue.

CHAPTER EIGHT

1. "Laetrile — An Answer to Cancer?" *Prevention*, December 1971.
2. James W. Sayre, M.D., and Sukru Kaymakcalan, "Hazards to Health: Cyanide Poisoning From Apricot Seeds among Children in Central Turkey," *New England Journal of Medicine*, May 21, 1964.
3. Renee Taylor, *Hunza Health Secrets* (New York: Award Books, 1969).
4. Copy of letter with the author.
5. *Berkeley Daily Gazette*, November 3, 1973.
6. Copy of letter with the author.
7. Herbert M. Summa, "Amygdalin, A Physiologically Active Therapeutic Agent in Malignancies," *Krebsgeschehen* 4 (1972).

CHAPTER NINE

1. Vilhalmur Stefansson, *Cancer: Disease of Civilization* (New York: Hill & Wang, 1960), p. 72.
2. Ernst T. Krebs, Jr., "The Nitrilosides in Plants and Animals," in *The Laetriles — Nitrilosides — in the Prevention and Control of Cancer* (Sausalito, California: Mc-Naughton Foundation, CA 1967).
3. Concretely, suggests Krebs, the following should provide 300 milligrams per day of vitamin B-17, if adhered to with some consistency.
   Breakfast—Gruel of buckwheat, millet and flaxseed, with elderberry jelly on millet toast, all of this accompanied by stewed apricots.
   Lunch—Lima beans or a succotash with chick peas; millet rolls with plum jam; elderberry wine.
   Dinner—A salad with bean and millet sprouts; dinner rolls of buckwheat and millet sweetened with sorghum molasses extracted from sorghum cane; rabbit which, one hopes, fed on clover; an after-dinner apricot, peach, cherry, or plum brandy originally prepared from crushing the whole fruit.
4. David M. Greenberg, Ph.D., "The Vitamin Fraud in Cancer Quackery," *The Western Journal of Medicine*, April 1975.
5. Dean Burk, Ph.D., *A Brief on Foods and Vitamins*. Sausalito, CA: The McNaughton Foundation, 1975.
6. Robert G. Houston "Sickle Cell Anemia and Dietary Precursors of Thiocyanate," Foundation for Mind Research, Pomona, N.Y., 1973. (An abstract of this paper appeared in the November 1973 *American Journal of Clinical Nutrition*.)

7. Houston strengthened the case for B-17 both in preventing sickle-cell anemia crisis and in association with extremely low rates of cancer in "Sickle Cell Anemia and Vitamin B-17 — A Preventive Model," *American Laboratory*, 7 (10):51-64, 1975. Administration of the simple chemical sodium cyanate (*i.e.*, an "outside" cyanate in contrast with an "inside" cyanate which could be a breakdown product of vitamin B-17 for relief in sickle-cell anemia was explored by Anthony Cerami and Charles M. Peterson in "Cyanate and Sickle-Cell Disease," *Science*, April 1975.

8. Stewart M. Jones, "The Immoral Banning of Vitamin B-17: How It Came About and How It Is Continuing." Palo Alto, California, January 1974.

CHAPTER TEN

1. Manuel D. Navarro, "Why Are Cancer Patients 'Pregnant'?," *Santo Tomas Journal of Medicine* 26. no. 3 (May-June 1971).

2. J. E. Dailey and P. M. Marcuse, "Gonadotropin Secreting Giant Cell Carcinoma of the Lung," *Cancer*, 24:388-396, August 1969.

3. Braunstein et al., *National Institutes of Health*, July 1973, quoted in *Physician's Handbook of Vitamin B-17 Therapy*, The McNaughton Foundation, P.O. Box B-17, San Ysidro, California, October 1973.

4. *Diagnosis of Cancer with Anthrone Test*, California Department of Public Health, 1964.

5. D. H. Koobs, "Phosphate Mediation of the Crabtree and Pasteur Effects," *Science* (October 17, 1972).

6. S. M. Jones, *Nutrition Rudiments in Cancer* (Palo Alto, Calif., 1972).

CHAPTER ELEVEN

1. Cited in Alan Stang, "Laetrile: Freedom of Choice in Cancer Therapy?" *American Opinion*, January 1974.

2. Dr. Burk's letter to Rep. Louis Frey, Jr., circulated both privately and published in *Cancer Control Journal*, May-June 1973, quoted NCI Director Dr. Frank Rauscher, Jr.: "Of the 100 cancers that afflict man, about fifteen percent of these can be treated extremely well, to the point of at least fifty percent five-year survivals." Burk extrapolated: 15% x 50% = 7.5%. I approached both NCI and American Cancer Society (ACS) spokesmen at the March 1974 ACS science writers' seminar on the above subject. Their consensus was that survival rates are indeed low — too low — but as of 1974 they thought it "dangerous" to make an across-the-board determination of 7.5 percent.

3. *Ibid.*

4. Letter, Dean Burk to Rep. Louis Frey, Jr., May 30, 1972, reported in *Cancer Control Journal* (May-June 1973).

5. Letter, Dean Burk to Hon. Robert A. Roe, July 3, 1973.

6. "Pulling Cancer's Energy Plug," *Medical World News*, October 9, 1973.

7. Burk and Dr. John Yiamouyiannis of the National Health Federation released a study claiming that 25,000 U.S. cancer deaths per year of 360,000 (the 1975 rate) were attributable to the fact the victims lived in areas with fluoridated water. The outcry, seconded by Rep. James J. Delaney, led to a congressional promise for a careful look at the possible fluoridation-cancer link as part of the examination, in 1977, of the National Cancer program.

CHAPTER TWELVE

1. Terri Schultz with Bard Lindeman, "The Victimizing of Desperate Cancer Patients," *Today's Health*, November 1973.

2. The stated Advisory Board as of 1971 was composed of Prof. N. R. Bouziane, M.D., Ph.D., director, research laboratories, Saint Jeanne D'Arc Hospital, Montreal; Senator David A. Croll, former minister of welfare and labor, Ontario; Charles Gurchot, Ph.D., pharmacologist involved in cancer research since 1931; Dr. James D. Hamilton, B.Sc., M.A., Ph.D., M.D., connected with two Montreal hospitals; R. T. Hewitt, O.B.E., M.A., secretary, Royal Society of Medicine, England; R. W. Howe, consulting engineer; Ernst T. Krebs, Jr., biochemist; Dr. Chauncey D. Leake, pharmacologist; Dr. Manuel D. Navarro, M.D., F.P.C.P., oncologist, Manila; Dr. Hans A. Nieper, internal medicine specialist, Hannover, West Germany; Dr. Fedor Romashov, professor of surgery, Lumumba University of Peoples Friendship, Moscow; Dr. Fedor Trinus, professor of pharmacology, Ministry of Public Health, Ukraine; Prof. Manfred von Ardenne, president, Manfred von Ardenne Research Institute, Dresden-Weisser Hirsch, East Germany.

3. "Emotions May Cause Cancer," *The San Francisco Chronicle*, June 9, 1976. (Associated Press article.)

CHAPTER FOURTEEN

1. *Physicians' Handbook of Vitamin B-17 Therapy*. McNaughton Foundation, San Ysidro, Calif., 1973.

2. *Ibid.*, p. 22

3. Barbara J. Culliton, "Sloan-Kettering: The Trials of an Apricot Pit — 1973," *Science* (December 1, 1973).

4. *Physician's Handbook of Vitamin B-17 Therapy*, p. 18.

CHAPTER FIFTEEN

1. Leo Levi, W. N. French, I. J. Bickis, and I. W. D. Henderson, "Laetrile: A Study of Its Physicochemical and Biochemical Properties," *Canadian Medical Association Journal* 92 (May 15, 1965): 1057-61.

APPENDIX I

How to answer the attacks by the American Cancer Society, the Food and Drug Administration, and local medical boards, against Laetrile (vitamin B-17)

The following is a primer on how to rebut the enormous propaganda campaign which has been mounted against Laetrile. The language used in the allegations is taken from statements made officially or informally by representatives of the above.

1. **Allegation: Laetrile is promoted as a mysterious cancer cure-all.**

Not true on any count. First, Laetrile is not promoted as a *cure* for cancer, let alone a cure-*all*. It is at best a *control* for cancer, and now is regarded as a metabolic agent or vitamin used in nutritional therapy and prevention. Second, Laetrile is not mysterious. The natural chemical amygdalin was isolated in its pure form in 1830. Its chemical structure has been known since that time. The extraction process of amygdalin from apricot kernels into the product Laetrile (injectable or tablet) is neither complicated nor mysterious.

Laetrile-using physicians around the world believe Laetrile, whether it directly kills cancer cells or not, provides noticeable relief for cancer patients. A majority of Laetrile-treated patients report positive responses, ranging from an increase in the feeling of well-being and even a brighter outlook on life, to such noticeable reactions as an increase in appetite, weight gain and, frequently, restoration of natural color, reduction or elimination of cancer-connected pain and of cancer-caused fetor. In a small but growing percentage of cases, total regression of all cancer symptoms has been confirmed.

The best effects from Laetrile use seem to be when it is used as part of a basic nutritional or metabolic therapy which also involves the administration of other vitamins, certain enzymes, and a diet from which animal protein has been mostly removed.

2. Allegation: Laetrile use is quackery.

Certainly *not* in any dictionary definition of the word ("fraudulent or ignorant pretense to medical skill"). The horrendous cancer rates under "orthodox" methods suggest who the *real* quacks may be. Many vital scientific and medical breakthroughs have been made by people who, in their day, were thought to be quacks. If Laetrile is quackery, then the Krebses and other vitamin B-17 pioneers are in pretty good company: Galileo, Pasteur, Lister, Semmelweiss, and Fleming for starters.

3. Allegation: Laetrile use is a cruel hoax in which conmen and hustlers are ripping off desperate cancer patients.

There may be scattered abuses by unprincipled people selling or offering Laetrile for sale. But this occurs *only* because the "establishment" continues to make Laetrile illegal. The situation is similar to the era of Prohibition: abuse of the populace, even introduction of poisonous material, an open door for organized crime — all these occurred *because* of government action. Any abuse in the Laetrile movement may be laid directly at the door of government.

The Laetrile recovery rates, testimonials, and growing positive-response statistics put the lie to the concept that Laetrile is a hoax — cruel or otherwise. Laetrile treatment in this country (involving merchandise sometimes bought from the black market) represents a cancer treatment almost always cheaper than "orthodox" treatment. And as for the two major Tijuana, Mexico, clinics constituting "ripoffs" — as of 1976, a three-week stay at either one characteristically cost from $1,000 to $3,000, a price normally including all room and board, a supply of take-home medicine, and, frequently, the roundtrip ticket to get there. This should be contrasted with a "normal" $15,000 to $20,000 price tag for "terminal" cancer sufferers in the United States, many of whom spend up to $50,000 before death ensues. The cancer industry's profits from drugs, radiation, surgical fees, insurance, hospital rooms, tests, checkups, internal medicine, anesthesia, etc. (all connected with cancer) may reasonably be set, as of 1976, at about $20 *billion* per year.

4. Allegation: Proponents of Laetrile are spreading false hope.

We *are* guilty of spreading hope. We know it isn't *false* hope. But even if it were, *false* hope would be better than no hope at all, which was all most "terminal" cancer patients in the United States were getting as of 1976.

5. Allegation: Spending time and funds on Laetrile is evil because it keeps cancer patients from useful orthodox treatments which might save them.

Hardly. The cancer institutions, cancer researchers, and statistical investigators referred to in this book provide the best evidence why this is not true. Survival rates from cancer in the U.S. have hardly improved since the 1950s, and, excluding skin and uterine cervical cancer, the *broad* statistical picture confirms "orthodoxy's" failure to stem the cancer pandemic through cutting, burning, and poisoning. One researcher has already shown that, *statistically,* a person with cancer is apt to live longer and feel better if he does *nothing at all,* rather than submit to surgery, chemotherapy and radiation.

6. Allegation: Testimonials don't mean anything. If you Laetrile people seem to have some it means that either the persons in question were misdiagnosed in the first place, are responding belatedly to orthodox treatment, or have undergone spontaneous remission. A lot of people subjectively feel better even with a sugar pill.

Nonsense. Of the now thousands of case histories, with the great majority of them showing *original diagnosis* in the United States, either more doctors than ever before are lying or are incompetent *or* they are diagnosing cancer. While in many cases "orthodox" treatment *has* — usually unsuccessfully — preceded the "Laetrile connection," it is no more scientifically appropriate to ascribe belated positive reactions to the earlier treatments than it is to claim the results are due solely to Laetrile.

As to those people who have been diagnosed in the U.S., and who underwent *only* Laetrile and its ancillary therapy, and have been found to be free of all symptoms, the phrase "spontaneous remission" can only be described as a "copout." As to "subjective feelings" based on sugar pills (placebos), the Laetrile-treated domesticated cats and dogs with cancer either are (a) psychic, (b) understand English, or (c) really do feel better.

7. Allegation: Laetrile has consistently been tested and retested without a shred of evidence as to its efficacy — not a sign of efficacy has been found.

No, no, a thousand times no! Part of such statements *may* be attributable to misleading criteria applied in animal studies, but mostly such statements are either ignorant remarks based on a lack of knowledge or, when uttered at the very top level of "orthodoxy" and bureaucracy, they are outright lies.

ANIMAL STUDIES: *SCIND Laboratories,* University of San Francisco, 1968, in which 400 rats bearing Walker 256 carcinoma (200 treated, 200 controls) showed up to 80 percent increased life spans at optimum dosages. *Pasteur Institute,* 1971, Paris. Increased life spans and delayed tumor growths noted in mice with human cancer strain; optimal dosage of 500 mg. Amygdalin Marsan per kilogram of body weight per day. *Institute von Ardenne*, Dresden, Germany, 1973. Increased life spans and decreased tumor growth noted in H-strain mice bearing Ehrlich ascites carcinoma treated with bitter almond amygdalin *ad libitum*, in addition to regular chow diet. *Sloan-Kettering Cancer Center*, New York, 1972-1975. In seven sets of data on experiments carried out by the famed Dr. Kanematsu Sugiura on mice specially bred to develop specific tumor systems, Laetrile was active in inhibition of the formation of lung metastases, inhibition in the growth of primary tumors, and in better health and appearance of the animals; in some other collaborative studies Laetrile was the implicit reason for life extension of test animals even when tumor growth was not slowed. The complete data from all of S-K's tests were not published when this was written, but the contradictory statements of S-K personnel and the results of authentic but "leaked" data are the strongest possible demonstration of a "shred of evidence . . . a sign of efficacy" from Laetrile use in animal studies. *Southern Research Institute*, Birmingham, Ala., 1974. Despite what "orthodoxy" *says* these data show, increased life spans were noted in a majority of 280 BDF1 mice bearing Lewis lung cancers treated with up to 400 mg. crystalline amygdalin per kilogram of body weight.

HUMAN STUDIES: While the thousands of case histories of use by humans in the United States, Canada, West Germany, the Philippines and several other countries *should* suffice to provide any rational mind with a "shred of evidence . . . a sign of efficacy," early test cases in published reports range from international and Italian medical journals in 1955 and 1958 (Guidetti and Tasca — see bibliography in this book) to American Dr. John A. Morrone's description of 10 cases in *Experimental Medicine and Surgery* (1962) and a gathering of much more human documentation in the McNaughton Foundation IND application of 1970, an application first granted, then suddenly yanked. The Guidetti, Tasca, Morrone data, and that of Dr. N R. Bouziane in Canada, and the additional data in the McNaughton Foundation IND, constitute several pounds of human test studies from the early era of Laetrile research.

8. Allegation: You cannot produce even one medically substantiated case which shows any beneficial effects.

Gasp! As of 1976, there were upwards of 6,000 "shreds of evidence" from the caseload of Dr. John A. Richardson, a carefully researched 4,800 cases by Mexico's Dr. Ernesto Contreras (culled from some 10,000 medical records developed by him in 14 years experience with Laetrile), almost 4,000 cases of total metabolic treatment by Dr. E. Paul Wedel of Oregon, himself a Laetrile recovery patient; 1,000 cases documented by Dr. Manuel D. Navarro, University of Santo Tomas, Manila, Philippines; a cluster of 100 Mexican government-monitored cases under the guidance of Dr. Mario Soto de Leon, medical director at the new Cydel Clinic, Tijuana, Mexico; additional hundreds treated by Dr. Hans Nieper, West Germany; and hundreds more being treated by a growing group of Laetrile-using physicians in the United States, including the records of such cancer victims as Glen Rutherford, Kansas, whose total recovery by Laetrile therapy at Tijuana is described in court records as a "cure."

All of the above are not triumphs for Laetrile, but many of them are. To claim these medical men (and the Indonesian researchers who claimed thousands of positive cancer responses to B-17 therapy from cassava) are all self-deluded or criminal or simply incompetent is the grossest kind of lie.

It's true that thorough documentation is hard to come by. Many major American hospitals and clinics will *not* release pathology reports to patients they know to be heading for Tijuana treatment centers. And, following the arrest of doctors in California and pressure brought on others in other states by their local medical boards because they dare to use "unproven" remedies in cancer, not too many medics are queuing up offering documented evidence of their treatment of patients with vitamin B-17.

9. Allegation: Eating seeds and kernels is dangerous because of the cyanide content.

It is true that eating *too many* B-17 natural foods will produce side effects, and that, at some biologically absurd point, perhaps even cyanide toxicity (as the Egyptians knew when they used the "apricot death" on prisoners). But too much of *anything* will produce dangerous side effects, including a thimbleful of water in the lung or a bubble of air in a vein. Under appropriate conditions, even gelatin, roast beef, and lettuce may release hydrogen cyanide. No one has (yet) attempted to control these foods, or even to stamp "Danger: Contains Cyanide" on American apples, each of which contains vitamin B-17-laden seeds. The *reductio ad absurdum* of the warnings about, and crackdowns on, apricot and peach kernels, will be confiscations of garbanzos, mung beans, buckwheat pancakes, sacks of millet, and prune, pear and cherry seeds, and possibly the removal of all nitrilosidic grazing grasses, since some human, somewhere, might choose to eat an acre or so of Johnson grass.

10. Allegation: Laetrile must be quackery because Dr. Krebs' degrees are honorary and Andrew McNaughton had an association with the Mafia and was a gunrunner.

Horsefeathers. The two Ernst T. Krebses, Sr. (an MD) and Jr., qualify as innovative scientists in the finest tradition. Krebs, Jr.'s writings, inventions, theories, patents and citations in medical literature qualify him as a scientist of the first magnitude, with or without "un-honorary" degrees. The story of Andrew R. L. McNaughton, an incredibly fascinating individual who was primarily responsible for keeping the Laetrile movement alive when it was on the way to being crushed out of existence by the "establishment," is told in this book. Readers may judge for themselves about McNaughton. But to attempt to destroy the theory and practice of Laetrile or vitamin B-17 by *ad hominem* attacks is a cheap shot.

11. Allegation: The Laetrile movement is connected with the John Birch Society.

Utterly ridiculous. Andrew McNaughton, the worldwide "Mr. Laetrile," who is also an honorary citizen of Cuba, can hardly be described as a "Bircher." Support for the concept of freedom of choice in medical therapy, and the fight for the vindication of Laetrile, has come from *all* shades of the political spectrum, and transcends ideology.

It's true that an impressive number of members of the JBS did become active in the Committee for Freedom of Choice in Cancer Therapy, Inc., because such Birchers, like many other individuals, believe and will fight for the concept of freedom of choice as an issue of more importance than Laetrile itself. For the record, there is NO official connection between the Committee and the JBS. There are Lions Club members, Pasadena Republicans, Detroit Democrats, self-described Communists, various rightists, a veritable horde of hip young people, and all kinds of others involved in the Laetrile movement. The "orthodox" opposition has accused the movement of just about everything except wife-beating and child-molesting, but there probably are a few of these persons who want to see cancer defeated, too.

12. Allegation: A lot of doctors are making money from Laetrile — and so are the smugglers.

The fact is, a lot of doctors are making money, *period*. You can bet your bottom dollar that those medics using "orthodox" 5-Fu, cyclophosphamide, methotrexate, radiation and similar horrors are making more than the gutsy physicians who use vitamin B-17 — but since when did the profit motive itself become a crime? As to the smugglers — again, while *some* abuses may occur, these are due to the government's unwritten ban and *de facto* illegalization of Laetrile.

The normal underground distribution in the U.S. of *Mexican* Laetrile (as of 1976 the most common and "purest" variety used in North America) included a 10-percent markup over the price of the products officially set by the Mexican government. This 10-percent markup, when weighed against the costs of transportation and distribution and the staggering legal fees for those people caught in the toils of the law because of involvement with B-17, hardly leaves much room for huge illicit profits. Naturally, distributors of vitamin B-17 (like distributors of aspirin and cough drops) seek to make a profit on their investment.

13. Allegation: If Laetrile proponents really have something, why don't they go through the usual licensing procedures like everyone else?

First, the well-intentioned 1962 Amendment to the federal Food, Drug and Cosmetic Act has made it awesomely complicated and expensive to license "new drugs," since both safety *and* efficacy must be demonstrated. This Amendment alone has caused a severe lag between the United States and many other advanced countries in the production of needed medical entities.

Second, the McNaughton Foundation, a non-profit organization, did make the attempt to secure an IND (Investigational New Drug license) in 1970. The IND was first issued — on the basis of an excellently documented submission by the Foundation. But it was suddenly withdrawn, less than two weeks later, because of "deficiencies" claimed in the original submission. Although the Foundation submitted the required additional data *within the specified time*, the Food and Drug Administration claimed it had not. This strange switcheroo fueled the "paranoid" suspicions of the laetrilists that the item would never get a fair hearing.

Third, inasmuch as amygdalin is a natural chemical, which was discovered in 1830 and therapeutically used less than a decade later, and inasmuch as even the modern extracted form of amygdalin as Laetrile had been in use well before 1962, laetrilists believe the substance has been "grandfathered." Moreover, they hold it is a food substance or vitamin and not a drug, either "new" or "old," and therefore should not be susceptible to control by the FDA.

Fourth, and perhaps the most important of all, the FDA guidelines for new drug licensing are specifically designed for companies or corporations which have a *proprietary interest* in a product. Since amygdalin is in the public domain and there is no patent on a vitamin, no company could hope to recover the huge investment required to license a vitamin. How much is involved in licensing a "new drug" under current guidelines? The best estimate in 1976 was that *at least* 5 to 10 years of animal studies would be needed, along with an expenditure of about $15 million and the completion of 80,000 pieces of paperwork.

The facts are that Laetrile is and has been in the public domain for a long time, it has been in general use among cancer patients, and it is a natural food substance for which no patent is outstanding (the only existing one, for freeze-drying, is now irrelevant since freeze-drying is no longer part of the production process). Because no investment in attempting to license a vitamin is likely to be recoverable, and also because it is doubtful that establishment forces would deal with Laetrile any more honestly now than in 1970, are reasons why the laetrilists don't "go through the usual licensing procedures." This point of view was shared by Western Oklahoma U.S. District Court Judge Luther Bohanon, who by 1976 had issued 18 court orders allowing terminal cancer patients to receive Laetrile supplies unhindered by the FDA, since, as he ruled, the FDA has "abdicated its responsibility" in the matter.

14. Allegation: Laetrile is illegal.

There is no federal law against Laetile, nor does Laetrile appear on an official list of proscribed items. The State of California has specific laws against the use of Laetrile for *human cancer*, as long as cancer is defined as a "space-occupying new growth" or neoplasm. A number of other states make the use of Laetrile in *cancer* indirectly "illegal" by giving cancer advisory committees the power to regulate the use of any remedies, proven or unproven. The Food and Drug Administration has used regulations, not law, to ban the interstate shipment and sale of Laetrile by alleging that it is either an "unlicensed new drug" or an "unsafe or adulterated food or food additive." Laetrile proponents argue that it is neither. Possession of Laetrile and private use by patients of Laetrile are not, in and of themselves, illegal.

The *de facto* (but certainly not *de jure*) "illegalization" of Laetrile springs from the FDA's regulatory ban, the specific California laws, and the pressure brought against physicians by state boards of medical examiners which control the licensing of such physicians. It is virtually as inappropriate to call Laetrile or vitamin B-17 illegal as it is to construe vitamin C or niacin as illegal. In California, despite the specific laws, the right of doctors to use vitamin B-17 as metabolic therapy, and without making specific claims as to "curing cancer," was established by court decisions in a number of cases.

APPENDIX II

Natural Sources of Vitamin B-17

Vitamin B-17 occurs abundantly in nature, but because of changes in our eating habits, and because of food processing, the normal Western diet is almost devoid of this vital food factor. Nonetheless, a diet in which vegetables and fruits play a central role will provide a certain amount of the substance, and any diet in which *whole fruits* and vegetables are consumed, including their seeds, is a guarantee of bringing *some* B-17 into the body. All fruits grown in North America *except* citrus fruits contain abundant portions of the vitamin in their seeds.

In the Western world, the highest concentrations of B-17 are to be found in the apricot and peach kernels, as well as in cherry seeds and in bitter (but not sweet) almonds. The following list of fruits, vegetables, grasses and grains is incomplete but represents common sources of the vitamin. Exact amounts of B-17 will vary depending on variety of plant, where grown and under what conditions.

KERNELS OR SEEDS OF FRUIT: The highest concentration of vitamin B-17 to be found in nature, aside from bitter almonds. Apple, apricot, cherry, nectarine, peach, pear, plum, prune.

BEANS: broad (Vicia faba), burma, chickpeas, lentils (sprouted), lima, mung (sprouted), Rangoon, scarlet runner.

NUTS: Bitter almond, macadamia, cashew.

BERRIES: Almost all wild berries. Blackberry, chokeberry, Christmas berry, cranberry, elderberry, raspberry, strawberry.

SEEDS: Chia, flax, sesame.

GRASSES: Acacia, alfalfa (sprouted), aquatic, Johnson, milkweed, Sudan, tunus, velvet, wheat grass, white clover.

GRAINS: oat groats, barley, brown rice, buckwheat groats, chia, flax, millet, rye, vetch, wheat berries.

MISCELLANEOUS: bamboo shoots, fuschia plant, sorghum, wild hydrangea, yew tree (needles, fresh leaves).

Two rules of thumb: While exact amounts of B-17 for a "minimum daily requirement" in cancer surveillance are not known, the basic concept is that sufficient daily B-17 may be obtained by following either of two suggestions:

First, eating all the B-17-containing fruits whole (seeds included), but not eating more of the seeds by themselves than you would be eating if you ate them in the whole fruit. *Example:* if you eat three apples a day, the seeds in the three apples are sufficient B-17. You would not eat a pound of apple seeds.

Second, one peach or apricot kernel per 10 lbs. of body weight is believed to be more than sufficient as a normal safeguard in cancer prevention, although precise numbers may vary from person to person in accordance with individual metabolism and dietary habits. A 170-lb. man, for example, might consume 17 apricot or peach kernels per day and receive a biologically reasonable amount of Vitamin B-17.

And two important notes: Certainly, you can consume too much of anything. Too many kernels or seeds, for example, can be expected to produce unpleasant side effects. These natural foods should be consumed in biologically rational amounts.

The highest concentrations of B-17 are obtained by eating the natural foods in their raw or sprouting stage. This does not mean that moderate cooking and other tampering will destroy the B-17 content. Foods cooked at a temperature sufficient for a Chinese dinner, for example, will not lose their B-17 content.

APPENDIX III

You Can Enjoy
Eating Vitamin B-17

While vitamin B-17 is characteristically bitter, and while consuming it in its highest concentrations in the natural form (apricot and peach kernels, bitter almonds) produces a bitterness which is generally repugnant to Western tastes, there is an infinity of ways to use vitamin B-17 in a palatable manner.

Seeds or kernels ground up in salads, or as part of salad dressing, or even served as a topping for ice cream (for those who do not avoid ice cream because of its high sugar content) are among ways to obtain natural B-17. Millet and buckwheat pancakes, elderberry jam, and even peach brandy prepared from crushing the whole fruit, are others.

The following recipes will provide you with many tasty ways to restore vitamin B-17 to your diet. *All* of these are indicated for use in the Laetrile diet for cancer patients, save in individual cases proscribed by doctors, and most include vitamin B-17 in its natural form.

CANCER DIET RECIPES

by Beverly Newkirk

The following recipes have been designed to accompany Laetrile (vitamin B-17) cancer therapy, unless specifically prohibited by doctors in certain cases. Most of them contain vitamin B-17 and may also be considered preventive recipes. No therapeutic claims of any kind are made or intended. We know these are tasty dishes, ideal for the patient on the Laetrile program.

In their preparation, only porcelain-coated iron or stainless steel containers should be used. Copperclad bottoms on stainless steel pots are all right, as copper helps to spread heat evenly. Remember, though, that copper utensils will destroy vitamin C on contact.

All vegetables in these recipes should be fresh. If this is not possible because of off-growing seasons in your part of the country, use vegetables that have been packed in glass — not metal — or frozen.

Some recipes call for mayonnaise — use homemade or buy at health food store.

GRAINS

Tabuli

1½ c. bulgar wheat	1 or 2 tomatoes, skinned, finely chopped
1 bunch parsley, minced	1 bunch mint
1 bunch green onions, minced	oil, lemon juice, salt

Soak the bulgar in cold water to cover for an hour or so until soft. Squeeze out the water with hands and mix with other ingredients. Dress with oil and lemon juice. Salt to taste. *It is important that vegetables be minced very finely.* Serve in a bowl surrounded with romaine leaves. The romaine is used to scoop up the Tabuli for eating.

Prepare the mixture a day early so that flavors blend well.

Millet with Herbs

1 c. millet	1 tsp. dried kelp
3 c. water	½ tsp. dill
½ small onion	1 tsp. basil

Place millet in 3 cups of water with ½ onion (do not chop or slice). Cover, cook about ½ hour. Watch millet closely so it does not over cook. It's best to do this ahead and let cool before continuing. Remove onion. Reheat millet in pan with 2 tbsp. oil. Add kelp, dill and basil.

SOUPS

Black Bean Soup

1 pt. black beans	2 qts. cold water
2 tbsp. chopped onion	1 hard cooked egg yolk
2 stalks celery, chopped	⅛ tsp. pepper
2 tsp. salt	½ tsp. dry mustard
2 cloves	1 tbsp. flour
	1 tbsp. margarine

Wash beans and soak overnight in water to cover. Drain and rinse. When ready to cook add onion, celery, salt and cloves, and cover with cold water. Boil slowly until beans are soft. Rub through a strainer. Add sufficient water to make the consistency of a thick cream. Mash the egg yolk with pepper and mustard and stir into soup mixture. Cook flour and margarine until a golden brown, thin with a little stock and stir into soup. Cook for 5 minutes, thinning with water if necessary.

Chicken Gumbo

1 small chicken, skinned	2 c. tomato pulp	1 c. diced celery
2 tbsp. flour	parsley	½ c. corn
1 onion, chopped	4 c. water	1 c. rice
4 c. okra, sliced or chopped	salt and pepper	
3 tbsp. margarine		

Clean chicken and cut into serving portions. Dredge lightly with flour and saute with onion in margarine. When chicken is browned, add okra, tomatoes, parsley, celery, corn, rice, and water. Season to taste with salt and pepper. Simmer until chicken is tender and okra is well cooked. Add water as needed during cooking. Serves 6.

Gazpacho

¾ c. finely chopped onion	¼ tsp. pepper
¾ tsp. minced garlic	1 tsp. paprika
1½ c. finely chopped green pepper	2 tbsp. chopped chives
2½ c. diced, peeled tomatoes	⅓ c. cold pressed oil
2½ tsp. salt	½ c. lemon juice
½ tsp. honey	2 c. tomato juice
	½ c. shredded cucumber

Combine onion, garlic, green pepper, tomatoes, salt, honey, pepper and paprika and chives in a large bowl. Stir in oil, lemon juice, and tomato juice. Chill 2 hours. Before serving blend in cucumber. 8 servings.

BREADS

Corn Bread

½ c. honey	¾ tsp. salt
2 eggs, beaten	1 c. stone ground cornmeal
2 c. millet flour	1 tbsp. cold press margarine
3 tsp. baking powder	1¼ c. soy milk

Mix honey and beaten eggs. Sift flour, baking powder and salt together and add to first mixture. Add cornmeal, melted margarine and milk. Beat just enough to mix. Bake at 400° for about 30 minutes.

Rye Crackers

½ c. water	1 c. millet flour
6 tbsp. oil	1 c. rye flour
½ tsp. salt	¼ c. sesame seeds

Mix well and knead. Let stand 10 minutes. Roll between two pieces of waxed paper until about ⅛″ thick. Score with knife into 1 inch squares. Bake 350° for 15 minutes.

DESSERTS

Fruity Freeze

1 lemon, peeled, seeded	½ banana, peeled
1 orange, peeled, seeded	3 tbsp. honey
½ c. pineapple, fresh or	4 ice cubes
unsweetened canned	

Blend all fruits and honey on high speed of blender. Add ice cubes gradually. Bits of orange peel may be added. Serve in chilled glasses.

Raisin Jumbos

2 c. raisins	½ tsp. cinnamon
¾ c. water	½ tsp. nutmeg
4 c. sifted millet flour	1 c. cold pressed margarine
1 tsp. baking powder	1 c. honey
1 tsp. soda	2 eggs, slightly beaten
1 tsp. salt	1 tsp. vanilla
½ c. chopped apricot or peach kernels	

Combine raisins and water and bring to boil. Boil about 3 minutes or until raisins are plump; cool. Sift flour, baking powder, soda, salt, and spices together. Cream margarine and honey together until light and fluffy; add eggs and vanilla and mix well; stir in raisins and any remaining liquid. Gradually add the flour mixture, blending thoroughly after each addition; stir in nuts. Drop by tbsp. one inch apart on greased cookie sheet. Bake 375° F. 12-15 min. Makes about 3 dozen cookies.

Flaky Pastry Shell

1 c. millet flour	¼ c. cold pressed oil
½ tsp. salt	2½ tbsp. ice water

Sift together flour and salt. Beat oil and ice water together with fork until creamy. Pour all at once over flour mixture and toss to form a moist dough. Form into ball, press into a flat round. Roll out between two pieces of waxed paper to fit pie dish. For baked pie crust cook at 475° F. for 10-12 minutes. Makes 9″ shell.

Date Tarts

1¼ c. dates, chopped	¼ c. apricot or peach kernels
½ C. orange juice	pastry

Combine dates, kernels and orange juice. Roll pastry ⅛″ thick and cut into rounds 3½″ in diameter. Place 1 tbsp. filling on each. Fold over, moisten edges and press together. Bake on ungreased cookie sheet at 450° F. 15 minutes. Makes 18.

Date Nuggets

1 c. wheat germ	2 tbsp. honey
1 c. pitted dates	1 tbsp. margarine
½ c. chopped nut meats	2 tsp. lemon juice

Put dates and nuts through food grinder. Mix with remaining ingredients. Shape into 1″ balls, chill. May be rolled in finely shredded coconut before chilling, if desired.

VEGETABLES

Brussel Sprouts with Lemon

1½ qts. brussel sprouts
¼ c. margarine
sea salt

pepper
lemon slices

Trim sprouts. Pour boiling salted water over them to cover. Let stand 5 minutes; drain. Melt butter in heavy skillet; add sprouts. Cover tightly and cook over very low heat just until they are tender, 10 to 20 minutes. Add salt and pepper to taste. Serve garnished with thin lemon slices.

Ratatoville

1 lb. eggplant
2 onions, sliced
oil
2 tomatoes, peeled

1 lb. zucchini
2 pimientos, cut into strips
minced garlic
assorted herbs and seasoning

Wash and dice eggplant. Brown sliced onion in oil; add tomatoes, zucchini, pimientos and eggplant. Add garlic and herbs to taste (oregano, basil and rosemary make a good combination). Simmer over low heat until vegetables are just tender.

Potato, Celery and Nut Loaf

¼ c. diced celery
¼ c. chopped nuts or apricot
    or peach kernels
3 c. mashed potatoes
3 tbsp. cold pressed margarine

1 egg, beaten
1 tsp. salt
⅛ tsp. paprika
2 tsp. grated onion

Cook celery until tender in small amount of boiling salted water. Drain off liquid. Add remaining ingredients in order listed. Mix well, pack in greased loaf pan and bake in moderate oven 350° F. for 35 minutes. Serves 6. May be served with tomato sauce.

Potato and Lima Bean Loaf

1⅓ c. cooked lima beans, mashed
⅓ tsp. sage
2 tsp. salt

4 tbsp. cold pressed margarine
½ c. soya milk
2 c. hot mashed potatoes

Mix lima beans with sage, 2 tbsp. margarine, 1 tsp. salt and ¼ c. soya milk. Place in bottom of a greased dish. Whip hot potatoes with remaining salt and milk and 1 tbsp. margarine. Place on top of lima bean mixture. Brush with remaining margarine. Bake at 425° F. for 15 minutes. Serve with tomato sauce.

Okra in Tomato Sauce

1½ lb. okra
1 small onion, sliced
3 tbsp. margarine
1¼ c. pulverized tomatoes

½ tsp. salt
⅛ tsp. pepper
3 tbsp. chopped parsley

Wash okra and cut off stems. Cut into ½" slices. Brown onion in margarine, add okra and cook about 5 minutes. Place in greased baking dish, add tomatoes, season and sprinkle with parsley. Bake at 350° F. for 30 minutes. Serves 6.

Corn and Celery

2 c. cooked corn	¼ tsp. salt
1½ c. diced celery	4 tbsp. margarine
½ c. minced ripe olives	½ c. soya milk
½ c. minced green olives	¼ c. dry bread crumbs
½ tsp. pepper	

Arrange corn, celery, olives and green pepper in alternate layers in greased baking dish. Add seasonings, 2 tbsp. margarine and soya milk. Cover with crumbs, dot with remaining cold-pressed margarine. Bake at 350° F. for 45 minutes. Serves 6.

Baked Carrots

18 small carrots	1 tsp. salt
⅓ c. margarine	⅓ tsp. cinnamon
¼ c. honey	⅓ c. boiling water

Scrape or pare carrots and place in casserole. Cream margarine and honey, salt and cinnamon together; add water and blend well. Pour over carrots, cover and bake at 350° F. for 1½ hours. Serves 6.

Beets in Orange Sauce

2 tbsp. butter	¼ tsp. salt
2 tbsp. cornstarch	¼ tsp. pepper
¾ c. water	2 tsp. honey
1½ tsp. grated orange rind	3½ c. sliced cooked beets
¼ c. orange juice	

Melt butter, stir in cornstarch and add water slowly. Add orange rind, orange juice, salt, pepper and honey. Cook until smooth and thickened, stirring constantly. Add beets, heat. Serves 8.

POULTRY AND SEAFOOD

Skillet, Apricot Chicken and Rice

1 chicken (3 lbs.) cut up	2 tbsp. oil
2 tbsp. flour	3 c. water
2 tsp. salt	1½ c. rice
¼ tsp. pepper	1 medium-size onion, sliced
½ tsp. leaf rosemary, crushed	1½ tsp. grated orange
¼ tsp. ground ginger	1½ c. dried apricots

Wash, dry and skin chicken pieces. Combine flour, salt, pepper, rosemary and ginger; dredge chicken in mixture; Heat oil in skillet, brown chicken pieces on all sides. Pour ½ C. water around chicken; cover and cook 15 minutes, adding more water if necessary. Push chicken to one side. Pour rice into pan, stir 1 minute to brown slightly. Add remaining ingredients; mix, cover; continue to cook 20 to 25 minutes or until rice is tender and liquid is absorbed. Serves 6.

Crunchy Chicken

½ c. potato starch
1 tsp. dried kelp
1 frying chicken (2½#) skinned
1 egg, slightly beaten

2 tbsp. water or soya milk
1 c. finely chopped apricot
kernels
2 tbsp. margarine, melted

Mix first two ingredients. Coat chicken. Dip in egg/water mixture. Coat with kernels and place on lightly oiled pan. Bake 375° for 30 minutes. Turn chicken and bake 30-40 minutes longer.

Sole Veronica

1½ c. water
1 c. white, unsweetened grape juice
¼ c. minced onion
1 bay leaf
3 or 4 whole peppercorns
(salt to taste)
2 lbs. fillet of sole
4 tbsp. each; margarine, flour

½ c. yogurt
1 tsp. lemon juice
½ tsp. Worcestershire sauce
pepper to taste
1 c. fresh seedless grapes
1 c. sliced mushrooms
paprika

Combine water, grape juice, onion, bay leaf, peppercorns and salt in a large heavy skillet; heat to simmering. Lay fillet of sole in liquid; cover and simmer 4 to 5 minutes or until fish is tender. Drain fillets, reserving liquids, and place in a greased shallow baking dish or an oven-proof platter. Strain reserved liquid; boil rapidly until reduced to ¾ cup. Melt butter and stir in flour; add yogurt and the ¾ c. fish liquid; cook, stirring constantly until mixture boils and thickens. Add lemon juice, Worcestershire sauce, salt and pepper. Stir in grapes and mushrooms. Pour hot sauce over fish, sprinkle with paprika. Place under preheated broiler 1 minute or until sauce is bubbly and delicate brown. Serves 5 or 6.

Chicken with Canton Sauce

1 chicken or duckling (5 lbs.)
   (skinned and cut in pieces)
¼ c. sliced green onions
⅛ tsp. pepper
3 tbsp. soy sauce
¼ c. cornstarch
3 tbsp. water
1 c. sliced mushrooms

3 eggs, beaten
½ c. water
1 c. flour
½ tsp. salt
oil
4 c. shredded lettuce
¼ c. sliced apricot or peach kernels

Place chicken in saucepan; cover with water. Bring to boil, reduce heat and simmer until chicken is tender. Drain. Reserve 2 cups fat-free broth.

In a small saucepan, combine reserved broth, green onions, pepper and soy sauce, bring to boil. Reduce heat and simmer 3 minutes. Blend together cornstarch and 3 tbsp. water until smooth. Stir into simmering mixture, add mushrooms and heat until clear; set aside and keep warm.

Combine beaten eggs, ½ c. water, flour and salt; beat until smooth. Remove meat from bones in large sections, cut into bite-size pieces; dip into batter. Drop pieces a few at a time into hot oil (375°). Fry until crisp and lightly brown.

Drain and place shredded lettuce on platter. Arrange chicken chunks in center, pour on hot sauce and sprinkle with sliced kernels.

Poached Salmon with Sauce Verte

5 qts. water
1 c. apple cider vinegar
¼ c. salt
4 carrots, sliced
2 large yellow onions, sliced
1 bay leaf

1 tsp. crumbled thyme
½ c. cooked chopped parsley
1 tbsp. peppercorns
1 fresh whole salmon (8-8½ lbs.)
cheesecloth

In a saucepan, combine water, vinegar, salt, carrots, onions, bay leaf, thyme and parsley. Bring to boil, lower heat and simmer 1 hour. Add peppercorn and simmer an additional 10 minutes. Strain into a large shallow pan big enough to hold the fish flat. Remove head and tail. Wrap salmon in cheesecloth 20″ longer than the fish. Put fish into broth and allow the long ends of cheese cloth to hang out of pan. Cover tightly, bring to a boil and then simmer for 30 minutes or until fish flakes easily. Remove lid and use the long ends of cheesecloth to lift the fish out of the pot. Put fish on a platter and carefully pull out the cheesecloth. Remove the skin and carefully remove the white fatty layer and the dark meat in the center of the fish. Serve with sauce verte and garnish.

Sauce Verte

1 tbsp. chopped capers, parsley,
cherries, watercress & tarragon
¼ c. water
1½ c. mayonnaise

1 tbsp. vinegar
3 drops tabasco sauce

Mix herbs and water and simmer for 5 minutes. Press mixture through a sieve. Cool. Stir mixture into mayonnaise with vinegar and tabasco sauce.

SALADS

Autumn Fruit Salad Bowl

1 head romaine
½ pineapple, pared & sliced
1 grapefuit, peeled & sectioned

½ red apple, sliced
¼ lb. red grapes
1 orange, peeled & sectioned

Line salad bowl with romaine. Divide bowl into 4 divisions with half slices of pineapple. Arrange alternate sections of grapefruit and apple slices in 1 division and place remaining fruits in separate divisions. Fill center with dressing. Serves 4.

Halibut Salad

3 c. cold cooked halibut
French dressing
1 cucumber, cubed
1 tbsp. chopped onion
Capers

1 tsp. salt
¼ tsp. pepper
mayonnaise
lettuce
pimiento

Flake the halibut in large pieces. Moisten with French dressing and chill thoroughly. Mix the halibut, cucumber, onion, salt and pepper with sufficient mayonnaise to hold the ingredients together. Serve on crisp lettuce leaves. Garnish with capers and pimientos. Serves 8.

Carrot-Raisin Salad

2 c. shredded carrots
½ c. raisins (unsulphured) or dates

½ c. wheat germ
½ c. mayonnaise

Mix ingredients together and serve on lettuce leaves.

Fruit Salad Bowl

1 bunch chicory
1 avocado, sliced lengthwise
3 bananas, cut into eighths
pineapple juice
3 slices pineapple,
cut into halves

6 plums, pitted
12 orange slices
6 wedges cantaloupe
18 watermelon balls
2 c. seedless grapes
dressing

Have ingredients well chilled. Arrange chicory in salad bowl. Dip avocado and bananas into pineapple juice to prevent discoloration; drain. Arrange fruit attractively on chicory, grouping all of each kind together. Serve with dressing arranging some of each fruit on individual plates. Serves 6.

Banana Salmon Salad

3 ripe bananas, diced
½ c. diced pineapple
1½ c. cooked salmon
mayonnaise to moisten

¼ c. diced celery
½ tsp. salt
1 tbsp. chopped pickle

Mix bananas and pineapple together. Add flaked salmon. Fold in remaining ingredients. Garnish with crisp lettuce or other greens and lemon slices. Serves 8.

Avocado Salad

3 avocados
1 c. pineapple cubes
1 c. grapes, halved
fresh mint

2 oranges, peeled & sectioned
French dressing
lettuce

Cut avocadoes into halves lengthwise and scoop out pulp. Save shells. Combine with other fruit and marinate in French dressing about 20 minutes. Fill avocado shells and serve on lettuce. Garnish with fresh mint. Serves 6.

Spring Salad Bowl

2 c. cooked or fresh uncooked
tender peas
6 raw cauliflowerets
2 c. cooked green beans
Radish roses

2 tomatoes
1 head lettuce
watercress
French dressing

Marinate vegetables seperately in French dressing and chill for 1 hour. Line salad bowl with outside leaves of lettuce and place 4 lettuce cups around center of bowl. Fill each with one of the vegetables and garnish center of bowl with watercress and radish roses. Serves 6.

Royal Salad

Lettuce
1 orange
1 grapefruit
dressing

1½ pears
1 green pepper
6 strawberries

Arrange lettuce on individual salad plates. On this arrange 3 segments of orange, 2 of grapefruit, 2 sections of pear, separating the different fruits with a slice of green pepper. Top with strawberry. Serves 6.

Papaya Salad

2½ c. diced papaya
1½ c. diced pineapple
1 c. sliced celery

¾ c. mayonnaise
2 tbsp. finely chopped onion
½ tsp. salt

Prepare fruit, combine with remaining ingredients, serve on crisp lettuce. Dress with mayonnaise and dash of paprika. Serves 8.

Grapefruit and Almond Salad

2½ c. grapefruit segments
1 c. shredded blanched almonds
½ c. chopped dates

1 green pepper, cut into rings
lettuce
dressings

Toss first 5 ingredients together and serve in lettuce cups. Serves 8.

Raw Cauliflower Salad

1 small head cauliflower,
thinly sliced
1 c. sliced celery
3 unpeeled red apples, diced
3 small green onions
¾ c. chopped parsley or
  1 bunch watercress, chopped

1 clove garlic
½ tsp. salt
¼ c. vinegar
¼ c. oil
pepper

Chill cauliflower, apples, celery, onions and parsley or watercress until very crisp. Rub salad bowl with garlic and salt. Serve with oil and vinegar.

Star Salad Bowl

1 c. sliced cooked beets
1 c. sliced cooked zucchini
1 c. sliced cooked gr. beans
1 c. sliced boiled potatoes
1 large head lettuce, shredded

2 hard-cooked eggs, chopped
1 c. French dressing
1 c. mayonnaise
6 ripe olives, chopped
2 hard-cooked eggs, sliced

Combine first 6 ingredients in salad bowl. Moisten with French dressing and a little mayonnaise. Cover top of salad with thin layer of mayonnaise. Arrange olives and egg slices on top. Serves 8.

Artichoke Salad

1 cooked artichoke per serving. Remove outside leaves and choke. Cut stems even so artichoke will stand straight. Fill centers with one of the following:

Mixture of leftover vegetables (e.g. beans, carrots, asparagus tips, peas, etc.) which have been marinated in French dressing, chopped hard-cooked egg, minced onion and chopped beets.

Serve with mayonnaise between artichoke leaves.

Bean Sprout and Water Chestnut Salad

2 c. sprouts (fresh)	¼ c. sliced water chestnuts
½ c. fresh pineapple, chunked	¼ c. slivered green pepper

Combine ingredients with following dressing:

1 c. mayonnaise	1 tsp. soy sauce
1 tsp. curry	

Sprinkle with ground or slivered apricot kernels.

SALAD DRESSINGS

Herbed Oil and Vinegar Dressing

¾ c. cold pressed oil	1 tsp. dry mustard
¼ c. natural apple cider vinegar	½ tsp. tarragon leaves
1 clove garlic	½ tsp. thyme leaves
1 tbsp. sorghum molasses	½ tsp. oregano leaves
1 tsp. sea salt	¼ tsp. pepper
1 tsp. paprika	

Mix together all ingredients. Chill several hours before using.

French Dressing

1 c. cold pressed oil	¼ tsp. white pepper
¼ c. apple cider vinegar	1 c. tomato juice
½ tsp. salt	½ clove garlic
few grains cayenne	1 tsp. honey

Combine and beat or shake thoroughly before using. Makes 2¼ cups.

BEVERAGE

Tea Punch

2 c. water, boiling	1 c. fresh lemon juice
2 tbsp. mint tea (herb)	1 c. fresh pineapple juice
½ c. honey	¼ c. Grenadine
3 c. fresh orange juice	1 qt. soda water

Combine water and tea. Steep for 10 minutes; strain. Add honey, fresh fruit juices and Grenadine and chill. Pour over ice block in punch bowl and stir in soda. Makes about 20 ½ c. servings.

APPETIZER

Avocado and Banana Kabobs

1 large, firm avocado
2 medium size bananas,
slightly green

1 large (not too ripe) papaya
lemon juice
honey

Peel avocado, bananas and papaya. Cut into ¼″ chunks. Brush with lemon juice, then with honey. Alternate on 12 hibachi sticks or skewers. Broil or grill 2 minutes on each side. Serve warm.

About the Committee for Freedom
of Choice in Cancer Therapy, Inc.

The Committee for Freedom of Choice in Cancer Therapy, Inc., was established in 1972 to fight for the right of doctors to practice without interference by the government; to educate the public about metabolic therapy, including vitamin B-17; to lead the fight for the recognition and legalization of nontoxic cancer therapy; to protect the doctor-patient relationship; and, in general, to battle for freedom of choice in therapy.

The Committee maintains a national doctor-patient referral service through which patients who seek metabolic therapy and physicians who use metabolic therapy, including vitamin B-17, in their practice, may be placed in contact.

The Committee also maintains a Physicians' Defense Group to help provide information and help for metabolic physicians whose allegiance to their Hippocratic Oath may have caused them problems with local medical boards or state authorities.

The Committee also operates as a national clearing house of information concerning vitamin B-17, non-toxic cancer therapy, and metabolic or holistic medicine.

The national headquarters invites interested readers to solicit more information and, if motivated, to help establish Committee chapters in their hometowns.

COMMITTEE FOR FREEDOM OF CHOICE
IN CANCER THERAPY, INC.
146 Main Street, Suite 408
Los Altos, California 94022
(415) 948-9475

BIBLIOGRAPHY

The following list of books, articles, and papers relating to Beardianism, vitamin B-17, the development of Laetrile, and related themes, is only partial. The entries were selected either for their thoroughness in telling the general story of vitamin B-17 or for their thoroughness in identifying key specifics in that area, or both.

BOOKS

Anatomy of a Coverup. Committee for Freedom of Choice in Cancer Therapy, Inc. Los Altos, California, 1975.

Bealle, Morris A. *Super Drug Story.* Washington: Columbia Publishing Co., 1962.

Beard, John. *The Enzyme Treatment of Cancer and Its Scientific Basis.* London: Chatto & Windus, 1911.

Burk, Dean, Ph.D. *A Brief on Foods and Vitamins.* Sausalito, California: The McNaughton Foundation, 1975.

Griffin, G. Edward. *World Without Cancer.* American Media, 1974.

Gurchot, Charles. *Biology — The Key to the Riddle of Cancer.* New York: Moore Publishers, 1949.

Kittler, Glenn D. *Laetrile — Control for Cancer.* New York: Paperback Library, 1963.

Stefansson, Vilhjalmur. *Cancer: Disease of Civilization.* New York: Hill & Wang, 1960.

Taylor, Renee. *Hunza Health Secrets.* New York: Award Books, 1969.

SCIENTIFIC ARTICLES, PAPERS, AND REPORTS

Brewer, A. Keith and Passwater, Richard. "Physics of the cell membrane; mechanisms involved in cancer," Part V. *American Laboratory* (April 1976).

Cerami, Anthony and Peterson, Charles M. "Cynate and Sickle-Cell Disease." *Science*, April 1975.

Contreras, Dr. Ernesto. *Reporte Preliminar: Comprendido de 500 Casos de Pacientes Tratados con Laetrile-Amigdalina.* Tijuana, Mexico (1967).

Dailey, J.E., and Marcuse, P.M. "Gonadotopin Secreting Giant Cell Carcinoma of the Lung." *Cancer* 24 (August 1969): 388-96

Diagnosis of Cancer with Anthrone Test. California Department of Public Health, 1964.

Greenberg, David M., Ph.D. "The Vitamin Fraud in Cancer Quackery," *The Western Journal of Medicine* (April 1975).

Guidetti, Ettore. "Observations Preliminaires sur Quelques Cas de Cancer Traites par un Glycuronoside Cyanogenetique." *Acta Unio Internationalis Contra Cancrum* 11 (1955): 156-58.

Gurchot, Charles. "The Trophoblast Theory of Cancer (John Beard, 1857-1924) Revisited." *Oncology* (Vol. 31, No. 5-6, 1975).

Houston, Robert G. "Sickle Cell Anemia and Dietary Precursors of Thiocyanate." Foundation for Mind Research, Pomona, N.Y., 1973. (An abstract appeared in *American Journal of Clinical Nutrition,* November 1973.)

———"Sickle Cell Anemia and Vitamin B-17 — A Preventative Model." *American Laboratory* (7 (10): 51-64, 1975).

Jones, Stewart M. *Nutrition Rudiments in Cancer.* Privately published, Palo Alto, California, 1972. (Distributed by Committee for Freedom of Choice in Cancer Therapy, Los Altos, California.)

Koobs, D.H. "Phosphate Mediation of the Crabtree and Pasteur Effects." *Science* (October 17, 1972).

Krebs, Ernst T., Jr. "The Nitrilosides in Plants and Animals." *The Laetriles — Nitrilosides — in the Prevention and Control of Cancer.* McNaughton Foundation, Sausalito, California, 1967.

———"The Nitrilosides (Vitamin B-17) — Their Nature, Occurrence and Metabolic Significance." *Journal of Applied Nutrition* 22, nos. 3, 4, (1970).

Krebs, Ernst T., Jr. and Bouziane, N.R. "Nitrilosides (Laetriles)." *The Laetriles — Nitrilosides — in the Prevention and Control of Cancer.* McNaughton Foundation, Sausalito, California, 1967.

Krebs, Ernst T., Jr.,: Krebs, Ernst T., Sr.,; and Beard, Howard H. "The Unitarian or Trophoblastic Thesis of Cancer." *Medical Record* (July 1950).

Lea, Koch, Morris. "Tumor-selective Inhibition of Incorporation of 3H-Labeled Amino Acids into Protein by Cyanate." *Cancer Research* (September 1975).

McCarty, Mark. "Burying Caesar: An Analysis of the Laetrile Problem." *Triton Times,* University of California at San Diego (Nov. 29, 1975).

Morrone, John A. "Chemotherapy of Inoperable Cancer (Preliminary Report of 10 Cases Treated with Laetrile)." *Experimental Medicine and Surgery* 4 (1962).

Navarro, Manuel D. "Biochemistry of Laetrile Therapy in Cancer." *Papyrus* 1 (1957): 8-9, 27-28.

———"Early Cancer Detection." *Journal of the Philippine Medical Association* 36 (1960): 425-32; and "Early Cancer Detection — A Biochemical Approach." *Santo Tomas Journal of Medicine* 15 (1960): 111-29.

———"Laetrile in Malignancy." *Santo Tomas Journal of Medicine* 10 (1955)

———"Laetrile — The Ideal Anti-Cancer Drug?" *Santo Tomas Journal of Medicine* 9 (1954): 468-71

———"Mechanism of Action and Therapeutic Effects of Laetrile in Cancer." *Journal of the Philippine Medical Association* 33 (1957): 620-27.

_____"Why Are Cancer Patients 'Pregnant'?" *Santo Tomas Journal of Medicine* 26, no. 3 (1971).

Physician's Handbook of Vitamin B-17 Therapy. McNaughton Foundation. Science Press International, P.O. Box 853, Sausalito, California, 1973.

Reitnauer, P.G. "Prolongation of Life in Tumor-Bearing Mice by Bitter Almonds." *Arch. Geschwulstforsch* 42, no. 4 (1974): 135-37 (East Germany).

"A Report on the Treatment of Cancer with Beta-Cyanogenetic Glucosides ('Laetriles')." California Department of Public Health (California Cancer Advisory Council), May 1963.

Sayre, James W., M.D., and Kaymakcalan. "Hazards to Health: Cyanide Poisoning from Apricot Seeds among Children in Central Turkey." *New England Journal of Medicine* (May 21, 1964).

Summa, Herbert M. "Amygdalin, A Physiologically Active Therapeutic Agent in Malignancies," *Krebsgeschehen* 4 (1972) (West Germany).

Summary of the McNaughton Foundation IND 6734 *(April 6, 1970-February 1971), Recent Case Histories, (and) the 'Grandfathering' of Laetrile-Amygdalin in the Treatment of Cancer.* McNaughton Foundation, P.O. Box 853, Sausalito, California, 1973.

Supplementary Report by the Cancer Advisory Council (State of California) on the Treatment of Cancer with Beta-Cyanogenetic Glucosides ("Laetriles"). Cancer Advisory Council, California Department of Public Health, 1965.

Tasca, Marco. "Observazioni Cliniche Sugli Effetti Terapeutici ci un Glicuronoside cianogenetico in Casi di Neoplasie Maligne Umane." *Gazzetta Medica Italiana, Edizioni Minerva Medica* (1958).

"The Treatment of Cancer with 'Laetriles'." *California Medicine* 78, no. 4 (April 1953).

"Unproven Methods of Cancer Management: Laetrile." *Ca-A Cancer Journal for Clinicians* 22, no. 4 (July-August 1972).

NEWSPAPER ARTICLES, MAGAZINE FEATURES, WIRE SERVICE ACCOUNTS, AND PUBLIC LETTERS

Bolen, Jean Shinoda. "Meditation and Psychotherapy in the Treatment of Cancer." *Psychic*, August 1973.

Burk, Dean. Letter to Frank Rauscher, Jr., director, National Cancer Institute, April 20, 1973.

_____ Letter to Rep. Louis Frey, Jr., May 30, 1972. *Cancer Control Journal* (May-June 1973).

_____ Letter to Rep. Robert A. Roe, July 3, 1973.

Culbert, Mike. "The Laetrile War Comes to Albany." series on Laetrile (vitamin B-17) *Berkeley Daily Gazette* and *Richmond Independent,* July 3-7, 1972.

Culliton, Barbara J. "Sloan-Kettering: The Trials of an Apricot Pit — 1973." *Science* (December 1, 1973).

Dean, Jim, and Martinez, Frank. "The Laetrile Story," series on vitamin B-17. *Santa Ana Register*, October 4-9, 1964.

"Debate over Laetrile." *Time*, April 12, 1971.

Drummond, William. "Cancer Victims Cross Border to Be Treated at Tijuana Clinics." *Los Angeles Times*, December 11, 1967.

"Emotions May Cause Cancer." *San Francisco Chronicle*, June 9, 1976.

Evans, M. Stanton. "Government Can be Hazardous to Your Health." *Imprimis*, Hillsdale College, Hillsdale, Mich., June 1975.

Gray, George. "FDA Blocks Tests of Anti-Cancer Vitamin." *College of Marin Times*, March 1, 1972.

Holles, Everett R. "Cancer Drug Smuggled into the USA." *Moneysworth*, May 10, 1976.

Jones, Stewart M. *The Immoral Banning of Vitamin B-17; How It Came About and How It Is Continuing*. Privately published, Palo Alto, California, 1974.

"Laetrile — An Answer to Cancer?" *Prevention*, December 1971.

Larson, Gena. "Is There an Anti-Cancer Food?" *Prevention*, April 1972.

Lyneis, Dick. "Cancer Victims Seek Tijuana 'Miracle'," two-part series on Laetrile (vitamin B-17). *Riverside* (Calif.) *Press*, April 25-26, 1972.

McCracken, Kenneth. Series on Laetrile (vitamin B-17). *Rochester* (Minn.) *Post-Bulletin*, January 21-25, 1974.

Matchan, Don C. "A New Look at Laetrile." *Let's Live*, June 1973.

Melnick, Norman. "Battle for a Banned Anti-Cancer Drug." *San Francisco Examiner*, July 4, 1972.

"Nation's Metabolic Experts Make Case for Legalization of California Chelation Therapy." *THE CHOICE*, May 1976.

"Pressuring the FDA on Laetrile," *Medical World News*, April 9, 1971.

Randal, Judith. "Unorthodoxy Given a Try." *Washington Star*, December 17, 1973.

Rorvik, David. "Laetrile: The Damn-Contraband-Apricot Connection," newsletter, The Alicia Patterson Foundation, New York, July 1976.

Ross, Walter S. "The Medicines We Need — But Can't Have." *Reader's Digest*, October 1973.

Schultz, Terri, with Lindeman, Bard. "The Victimizing of Desperate Cancer Patients." *Today's Health*, November 1973.

Stang, Alan. "Laetrile: Freedom of Choice in Cancer Therapy?" *American Opinion*, January 1974.

Sullivan, Brian, and Saltus, Richard. Two-part series on Laetrile (vitamin B-17). Associated Press, February 4-5, 1974.

Sullivan, Rick. "50 Peninsulans Using Vitamin to Treat Cancer." *Menlo-Atherton* (Calif.) *Recorder*, June 13, 1973.

Valentine, Tom. Three-part series on vitamin B-17 (Laetrile). *National Tattler*, March 11, 18, 25, 1973.

Von Hoffman, Nicholas. "And If It Works...." *Washington Post*, June 4, 1971.

Westover, Wynn, editor. *See the Patients Die* (essays by and about cancer patients and B-17). Science Press International (Box 855, Sausalito, California 94965), 1974.

"Will Laetrile ... Get the Legal Status of Another of Dr. Krebs' Discoveries...?" *Alameda* (Calif.) *Times-Star*, January 14, 1967.

INDEX

C

food processing - 135
Foundation for Mind Research - 143
Freedom Newspapers - 110
"freedom of choice" law, approved in
    Alaska - 26
Frey, Rep. Louis - 121, 158

G

Garland, Henry L. - 111
Geczy, Alex - 129
Gerson, Max - 76
Gibson, Bettie - 11
Gillespie, I. E. - 157
Glaser, Ralph - 161
glyoxylide - 76
Goenawan, Mas - 124, 138
Gold, Joseph - 161
Good, Robert A. - 23
Greenberg, Daniel - 15-16
Greenberg, David M. - 142
Griffin, G. Edward - 12, 79
Grosch, Margaret - 31
Guevara, Che - 169
Guidetti, Ettore - 111
Gurchot, Charles - 89, 91, 97, 99,
    100, 102, 178

H

Haldane, J. B. S. - 91
Hanson, Donald - 9
Harper, Harold - 177
Harris, Arthur T. - 108
Harrison, Steven - 174
Harvard Medical School - 19
HCG. *See*, chorionic gonadotropin
Hillyard, Raymond - 123
Hoffman, Herb - 174
Hoiles, Douglas - 175
Holland, James F. - 160
Houston, Robert G. - 143
Howard, Harvey E. - 111, 150
Hoxsey Cancer Clinic - 77
Hoxsey, Harry - 78
Huks, diet of - 137
Humphrey, Sen. Hubert H. - 26
Hunza Health Secrets -128
Hunzakuts - 128

Hutchinson, Jay - 22, 33, 63, 128
hydrazine sulfate - 154, 161
hydrogen cyanide - 106

I

Ilocano Filipinos - 137
IND. *See*, Investigative New Drug
    applications
Indian Doctor's Dispensatory, The - 85
Inosemtzeff, T. - 87
Institute of Nutritional Research -
    150
Internal Revenue Service - 31
International Association of Cancer
    Victims and Friends (IACVF) -
    13, 28, 36, 40
International Union Against Cancer -
    111
Investigative New Drug (IND) appli-
    cations - 113-115, 120-121
Ivy, Andrew C. - 76

J

Jane Roe v. *Henry Wade* - 37
John Beard Memorial Foundation -
    91
John Birch Society - 27, 30, 78, 81,
    84, 166, 170
Jones, Hardin B. - 17
Jones, Stewart M. - 11, 45, 144, 145,
    147, 166, 175
*Journal of the American Medical Asso-
    ciation* - 137, 140
Josephson, Emanuel M. - 82

K

Kell, George - 37, 26, 111
Kennedy, F. - 157
Khan, Prince Mohammed Ameen -
    129
Kilpatrick, James - 11
Kittler, Glenn - 96, 109
Koch, William S. - 76
Koobs, D. H. - 147
Krebiozen - 76-78
Krebs, Ernst T., Jr. - 35, 40, 43, 86,

Old, Lloyd J. - 42, 66, 179

P

pangametin. *See,* pangamic acid
pangamic acid - 118, 146, 164
Passwater, Richard A. - 105
Pauling, Linus - 24
Peters, Vera - 157
Physician's Handbook of Vitamin B-17 Therapy - 168
Powers, William - 156
Prevention - 60
preventive medicine - 80
Privitera, James - 11, 57, 68, 177
Proxmire Law - 29
Psychic - 167

R

Rauscher, Frank, Jr. - 67
Richards, Victor - 67, 155
Reader's Digest - 113
Review of the News, The - 175
Richardson, John A. - 11, 12, 27, 29, 30, 34, 64, 111, 123, 143, 151, 169, 170; arrested and tried, 30-32; defends Laetrile, 34-35; establishes clinic, 64
Robiquet, Pierre Jean - 87
Rochester (Minn.) *Post-Bulletin* - 11, 173, 190
Roe, Rep. Robert A. - 160
Rorvik, David M. - 42
Rosenberg, Saul A. - 157
Rubin, Philip - 157
Rutherford, Glen - 37, 47, 190

S

Salaman, Frank - 169-174
Salaman, Maureen - 174
San Francisco Vegetarian Society for Health and Humanity - 102
San Mateo County Medical Society - 149
Santo Tomas, University of - 145
Scarburgh, Charles - 73
Schepartz, Saul A. - 43
Schmid, Franz A. - 41

Schmidt, Alexander MacKay - 13, 21
Schmidt, Benno C. - 21, 38
Schuster, Donna - 9
Schweitzer, Albert - 76
Science - 147
Senate Interstate Commerce Committee on the Need for Investigation of Cancer Research Organizations - 77
Seventh-Day Adventists - 20, 46
sickle-cell anemia - 143-144
Simandjuntak, Todotua - 124, 138
Simonton, O. Carl - 167-168
Sittig, Charles W. - 53
Sixth National Cancer Conference - 156
Sloan-Kettering. *See,* Memorial Sloan-Kettering Cancer Center
Smith, Pat - 51
Sowinski, James W. - 54
Soto de Leon, Mario - 122
Stang, Alan - 57, 84
Stefansson, Vilhjalmur - 136
Steinbacher, John - 28
Steinfeld, Jesse - 120, 190
Stock, Chester - 39
Stockert, Elizabeth S. - 41
Sugiura, Kanematsu - 39-41, 65
Sullivan, Robert D. - 156
Summa, Herbert M. - 86, 131
Super Drug Story - 82
Sweet, Helen - 174
Sweigert, Judge W. T. - 112
Symms, Rep. Steven - 26

T

Tausog Muslims - 137
Taylor, Renee - 129
Test Laetrile Now Committee - 22, 32, 63
Thurston, Emory - 150
"Tijuana connection" - 30, 118
Today's Health - 166
Tornay, Stephen - 130
Trelford, John D. - 158
trophoblastic theory of cancer - 88, 90, 100, 103, 180

U

unitarian theory of cancer. *See*, trophoblastic theory of cancer
urine test for cancer - 111, 146
Urrutia, Manuel - 165

V

Vilcabamba Indians - 46
vitamin B-15. *See*, pangamic acid
vitamin B-17. *See*, Laetrile
*Vitamin B-17: Forbidden Weapon
   Against Cancer* - 12, 39
von Hoffman, Nicholas - 11
von Liebig - 87

W

Warburg, Otto - 154, 161
Wardell, William - 114
Watts, Clyde - 37, 48
Wayward Cell, The - 155

Wedel, E. Paul - 64, 123, 177
Weilerstein, Ralph - 127
Welsch, Clifford W. - 20
Werner, Ben - 127
Westover, Wynn - 96, 98
Who's Who in the World - 154
Wilkey - 85
Wilkinson, Joan - 60
Williams, Billy - 52-53
Winston, Frank - 33
Wohler, Friedrich - 87
World Without Cancer - 12, 79, 83
Wynder, Ernest L. - 20

Y

Young, Mort - 41

Z

Zalac, Stephen - 167
Zicarelli, Joseph (Bayonne Joe) - 170
Zubrod, C. Gordon - 44